Hypoglycemia
FOR
DUMMIES®
2ND EDITION

by Cheryl Chow
Writer and editor

by James Chow, MD
Practicing physician

BICENTENNIAL
1807
WILEY
2007
BICENTENNIAL

Wiley Publishing, Inc.

Hypoglycemia For Dummies®, 2nd Edition

Published by
Wiley Publishing, Inc.
111 River St.
Hoboken, NJ 07030-5774
www.wiley.com

For general information on our other products and services, please contact our Customer Care Department within the U.S. at 877-762-2974, outside the U.S. at 317-572-3993, or fax 317-572-4002.

For technical support, please visit www.wiley.com/techsupport.

Wiley also publishes its books in a variety of electronic formats. Some content that appears in print may not be available in electronic books.

Library of Congress Control Number: 2007920018

ISBN: 978-0-470-12170-2

Manufactured in the United States of America

10 9 8 7 6 5 4

WILEY

About the Authors

Cheryl Chow has been a freelance writer, editor, and journalist for more than 20 years, concentrating on health and social issues. She has a diverse writing background, having written for magazines, newspapers, webzines, and literary magazines. She and Dr. Chow have coauthored a reference book on hepatitis and other liver diseases.

Coming from a family with a long line of medical doctors, Chow has always been fascinated by medicine and science. After obtaining a BA in psychology from Reed College, she pursued her own studies into the effects of mind over body, and vice versa. She has conquered her own bouts with hypoglycemia, fatigue, and other health issues through attention to lifestyle and diet. She has studied T'ai Chi, chi kung, ba gua, and meditation from some world-renowned teachers, and has also taught T'ai Chi exercises for health.

James H. Chow, MD, is the founder, CEO, and medical director of multispecialty clinics offering integrative medicine and diverse treatment modalities located in New York, Westchester, Chicago, Atlanta, and San Diego. Dr. Chow specializes in emergency and family medicine. Before he went into private practice almost 20 years ago, he was the director of the emergency department at Mt. Sinai Hospital in Chicago for seven years. As an emergency doctor at one of the busiest hospitals in the U.S., he has encountered and treated almost every imaginable type of illness and injury. Dr. Chow is licensed to practice medicine in Illinois, Georgia, and New York. In 1996, Dr. Chow helped set up an American-style clinic in Beijing.

Dr. Chow is a member of American Academy of Emergency Medicine, American Academy of Physician Executives, American Academy of Sports Medicine, American Academy of General Medicine, American Academy of Family Practice, Nippon Industrial Medicine Association, and American Japanese Physicians Association. Having too much time on his hands, Dr. Chow is currently involved with various medical projects. He's known among his friends and associates for his unbounded energy, personal warmth, and sense of humor — had he not become a medical doctor, Dr. Chow could undoubtedly have become a comedian.

Dedication

We dedicate this book to our mother, who has inspired us with her indomitable spirit. Late in life she became a published novelist and essayist (with fan mail from all over the world). Always young at heart, most of her friends are half her age.

This book is also dedicated to our father, without whose foresight and financial support neither of us would have been blessed with the education and career opportunities that we have had.

Authors' Acknowledgments

I would like to thank everyone, especially the various healthcare practitioners whose knowledge, expertise, and experience helped shape this book. Thanks especially to Dr. Carolyn Dean, MD; Dr. Colleen Huber, NMD; Raymond Hinish, PharmD, CN; Dr. Michael T. Murray, ND; Dr. Iljong Kim, MD; and EFT founder Gary Craig for giving up their valuable time to answer my numerous questions. Dr. Huber in particular was more than generous in sharing her vast knowledge.

Special thanks and much gratitude also to John Hartsell for his expertise in wordsmithing and his critical eye for detail.

I would like to express my appreciation to my brother and coauthor, Dr. James Chow, for his share of the work, and for his gift of a MacBook, which was used in the writing of the manuscript. I also want to thank the staff of the Nihon Clinic. And last, but certainly not least, I want to thank my agent Elizabeth Frost-Knappman of New England Publishing Associates, and the staff at Wiley Publishing, in particular Michael Lewis, the acquisitions editor, Chad Sievers, the project editor, and Sarah Faulkner, the copy editor.

Publisher's Acknowledgments

We're proud of this book; please send us your comments through our Dummies online registration form located at www.dummies.com/register/.

Some of the people who helped bring this book to market include the following:

Acquisitions, Editorial, and Media Development

Project Editor: Chad R. Sievers

(Previous Edition: Tonya Maddox Cupp)

Acquisitions Editor: Michael Lewis

Copy Editor: Sarah Faulkner

(Previous Edition: Greg Pearson)

Technical Editor: Lorna Walker, PhD, nutritionist for the Hypoglycemia Support Foundation, Inc.

Editorial Manager: Michelle Hacker

Editorial Assistants: Erin Calligan Mooney, Joe Niesen, Leeann Harney

Cartoons: Rich Tennant (www.the5thwave.com)

Composition Services

Project Coordinator: Heather Kolter

Layout and Graphics: Carl Byers, LeAndra Hosier, Stephanie D. Jumper, Erin Zeltner

Anniversary Logo Design: Richard Pacifico

Proofreader: Aptara

Indexer: Aptara

Publishing and Editorial for Consumer Dummies

Diane Graves Steele, Vice President and Publisher, Consumer Dummies

Joyce Pepple, Acquisitions Director, Consumer Dummies

Kristin A. Cocks, Product Development Director, Consumer Dummies

Michael Spring, Vice President and Publisher, Travel

Kelly Regan, Editorial Director, Travel

Publishing for Technology Dummies

Andy Cummings, Vice President and Publisher, Dummies Technology/General User

Composition Services

Gerry Fahey, Vice President of Production Services

Debbie Stailey, Director of Composition Services

Contents at a Glance

Table of Contents

Introduction

*I*f you pick up this book, chances are you've been suffering from
the blues for a long time: the low blood sugar blues, that is. If
you're hypoglycemic, you know that you don't have to go to an
amusement park to experience the roller coaster effect; your blood
sugar does it for you automatically, thank you very much. In addition, you may often get the jitters (especially after a stretch of time
without food), and become nervous, edgy, and irritable. You're
chronically tired, and you wake up in the morning not feeling the
least bit rested. Or maybe you have other complaints, such as
depression, that just don't respond to medical treatments — or
any other remedies.

Your colleagues, friends, and family may be tired of your moods,
your chronic fatigue, and your various aches and illnesses, none of
which seems to have a clear, attributable cause. You've been to
many doctors. And what do they tell you? They tell you that all the
lab tests have come out "essentially negative." You're afraid that
the doctors regard you as neurotic or, at best, a hypochondriac. Or
perhaps you received a clear diagnosis. But now your real strug-
gles begin. No magic pills can instantly cure you.

The good news is that, with a better understanding of hypoglycemia
and the program of recovery outlined in this book, you can regain
your health, your wits, and your sense of humor. And who knows,
you may — depending on your genes and, aside from hypoglycemia,
whatever else may be going on with your body — appreciate life
more than many of your currently enviably healthier brethren.

About This Book

Since the first edition of *Hypoglycemia For Dummies* came out in
2002, many more studies have been published on how foods affect
your health. Although the basic hypoglycemia diet remains the
same, we know much more than we did about the effect of different
fats on the body. At the same time, more light has been cast on the
dangers of artificial sweeteners and monosodium glutamate (MSG).

When writing this second edition, we hope to provide you, our
readers, with the latest information on the subject of health and
diet. Thus, we expand many chapters, most noticeably Chapter 6,

which tells you what foods to eat and to avoid. You can find many suggestions on various food substitutes throughout the book; we also offer tips on how to make the transition to a hypoglycemic diet. We try to make the book as user-friendly as possible for the busy reader who's not only pressed for time, but also has health issues that may make it more difficult to read or to absorb new information.

Conventions Used in This Book

To make everything as easy as possible, we use the following basic conventions to help you:

- We *italicize* all medical terms and provide an immediate definition. We also attempt to explain any other words or concepts that may be difficult to understand or may be subject to misunderstanding.

- We use `monofont` to identify all Web sites and e-mail addresses.

- We **bold** all key words in bulleted lists and all the steps in numbered lists.

Furthermore, whenever we mention hypoglycemia, unless otherwise indicated (and we'll make that amply clear), we mean the hypoglycemia related to one's diet — the type that people refer to when they feel weak from low blood sugar. We use the word *recovery* because health is an ongoing process, not something that you can attain with a quick-fix approach. Your challenge is to correct not only the imbalances of your body but also the way you live, work, play, and relate to others.

What You're Not to Read

We have good news for you busy people! You don't have to read this book from cover to cover. Of course we want you to read everything, but we understand that you may want to read just the essential info. If that's the case, feel free to skip

- **The sidebars.** They're interesting info and appear in the little gray boxes, but they're not essential.

- **The Library of Congress info.** We're required by law to include this mumbo jumbo text, but it's not important to you.

Icons Used in This Book

The icons are signposts to help you identify what parts of the book are indispensable.

This icon indicates useful information about hypoglycemia. It can save you time, or money, if you're lucky.

The book has a lot of information, but this icon highlights the stuff that'll do you the most good.

This icon presents very important information that you should be aware of. Don't ignore this icon! Doing so may be detrimental.

Right, call the doctor! When you see this icon, you'll know that we recommend that you go see a physician.

Foolish Assumptions

If you pick up this book, we assume that you

- ✔ Suffer from symptoms associated with hypoglycemia (or someone close to you suffers from the symptoms) and you want to alleviate the symptoms

- ✔ Aren't a specialist in the medical field (You want just the basic essential info so you can better grasp your condition.)

- ✔ Are aware of the controversy surrounding this syndrome but accept — or at least suspect — that such a medical problem indeed exists

How This Book Is Organized

This book has five parts to make navigating easier. It's a handy reference for the busy person, because much of the relevant info is compiled together under one cover for your convenience.

Part I: Addressing Your Ups and Downs: Could This Be Hypoglycemia?

Part I addresses the most important facts about hypoglycemia. What causes it? Who's most susceptible? We talk about some of the hypoglycemic complications that may result from diabetes, as well as other common symptoms.

Part II: Diagnosing and Treating Your Hypoglycemia

This part helps you find a supportive doc who can help you determine whether you suffer from this condition. We sort through the complexities and permutations of this syndrome and rule out other possible causes for what's ailing you. We also discuss everyone's favorite subject: food. We explain the part that nutrition plays in everyone's health and the great significance it has for hypoglycemics. We give info on vitamins, herbs, and supplements.

Part III: Emulating Lifestyles of the Well and Healthy

This part maps out the lifestyle that can help you achieve the vibrant health you desire. We show you how to choose exercises that are fun and give tips on how to make your working life easier.

Part IV: Spinning a Network of Support for Yourself (and Others)

Because everyone needs the support of other people, in this part, we show you how to set up a support network, both online and offline. We also reach out to your loved ones and give them a little support.

Part V: The Part of Tens

Are you forever explaining hypoglycemia to people? This part gives you the straight facts on common myths and misperceptions about hypoglycemia. You want some help staying on the narrow and true diet path? You got it with tips and hints on what to do when temptation strikes.

Where to Go from Here

Feel free to turn to the section that seems most relevant to you and start reading. Where should you go? First, check out the table of contents and index to see what topics interest you the most. If you know nothing about hypoglycemia, start with Chapter 1, which gives you a brief overview, and Chapter 2, which gives you the nitty-gritty technical scoop. If you want the lowdown on food and diet, check out Chapter 6. If you suspect that someone close to you is hypoglycemic, start with Chapter 14. No matter where you go, you can find valuable info that can help ease this condition.

Part I

Addressing Your Ups and Downs: Could This Be Hypoglycemia?

The 5th Wave   By Rich Tennant

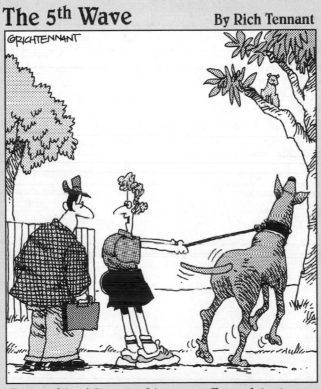

"I call him 'Glucose,' because I need to keep him under control every day."

In this part . . .

*I*f you want to know the most important facts about hypoglycemia, you can find them here. This part lists the different types of hypoglycemia that are known to the medical world, and how they may affect people at different ages. We cover some of the hypoglycemic complications that can result from diabetes, and we tell you about other common conditions that you should watch out for. We also show you just how many symptoms are associated with hypoglycemia.

Chapter 1

Riding the Blood Sugar Roller Coaster Isn't Any Fun

*O*ver the years, researchers have coined different names for the condition that people suffer from when they believe that they have hypoglycemia, including functional hypoglycemia, relative hypoglycemia, disinsulinism, hypoglycemic fatigue, and insulinogenic hypoglycemia. Don't get too hung up on the names, though. Your attention should be on regaining your health, not worrying about what your constellation of symptoms should be called.

No matter what you or your doctor calls your low blood sugar, this chapter is a great starting point. This chapter gives you the lowdown on hypoglycemia, who's prone to having it, and what you can do to make this roller coaster ride not so rough.

Defining Hypoglycemia

Defining hypoglycemia is easy. It's low *(hypo)* blood sugar *(glycemia)*. Modern medicine, or allopathic medicine, which is Western medicine as it's practiced in developed countries, recognizes two major categories of hypoglycemia — organic and fasting, which both generally have clear-cut causes — as legitimate. Other types of hypoglycemia, which fall under the category of relative and reactive hypoglycemia, aren't usually recognized by mainstream medicine. It's still a controversial subject, although some studies indicate that sensitive people can suffer from hypoglycemic-like symptoms even when their blood sugar doesn't drop to a level that's medically defined as hypoglycemia. (See Chapter 5 on how blood sugar is measured.)

The diagnosis of *idiopathic reactive hypoglycemia,* or *reactive hypoglycemia* for short, isn't universally accepted by allopathic doctors. This is the type of hypoglycemia that people are referring to when they complain of being hypoglycemic. Reactive hypoglycemia is also this book's focus. In the rest of this book, unless otherwise stated, we're talking about reactive hypoglycemia.

But before you get into the rest of the book, take a look at the following sections to discover more about the different types of hypoglycemia and see where your symptoms might fall.

Organic

With *organic* hypoglycemia, your blood sugar level when you've been fasting is invariably low. (The *fasting level* is the amount of sugar in your blood after *fasting* — not eating anything — for 10 to 12 hours.) The symptoms are usually continuous.

This type of hypoglycemia is very rare and may be caused by glandular defects or tumors. If you have organic hypoglycemia, it warrants further investigation to determine whether you have an enlarged pancreas, tumors of the pancreas, or other causes that are unrelated to what you do or don't eat.

Relative

Relative hypoglycemia is a condition where your blood sugar declines from an elevated level to a low level quite rapidly. The group of people most often misdiagnosed as normal suffer from relative hypoglycemia. For example, you're said to have relative hypoglycemia if

✔ Your blood sugar falls 20 milligrams (mg) or more below your fasting level within six hours after eating, and you experience symptoms.

✔ Your blood sugar falls 50 mg or more within one hour after eating, and you experience symptoms.

✔ During the test that checks your blood sugar level, your blood sugar increases by 20 mg or less after ingesting the glucose that you're given to drink for the test, and then falls to at least 20 mg below your fasting level. (Chapter 5 describes the test you can take to check your blood sugar level.)

Reactive

Reactive hypoglycemia refers to how your body reacts after you eat. How high or low does the blood sugar go? With this type of hypoglycemia, symptoms fluctuate according to the food you eat, the time of day when you eat, and so on. In reactive hypoglycemia, the level of sugar in your blood when you've been fasting may be normal or even a little above what's considered normal. Your body then overreacts to the glucose in the food you eat by producing too much insulin, which causes the fall in blood sugar. (That's why it's called *reactive*.) Even if the blood sugar doesn't fall below what's considered the normal range, a person may experience symptoms of hypoglycemia if the fall is fast enough.

Many health practitioners don't differentiate between reactive hypoglycemia and relative hypoglycemia. They lump the two together and call it *functional hypoglycemia*. If you hear this term, it refers to hypoglycemia that typically occurs because of an imbalance in the body chemistry, probably due to an overactive pancreas producing too much insulin.

Fasting hypoglycemia is sometimes classified as being part of functional hypoglycemia. It can occur when you haven't eaten for a while. How long that is depends on the individual, but it's generally several hours after a meal.

If your doctor uses the term *idiopathic postprandial reactive hypoglycemia* or *idiopathic reactive hypoglycemia,* he's talking about reactive hypoglycemia. *Idiopathic* is just a fancy word that doctors use to say, "We haven't got a clue what causes it." (Now you know how to profess ignorance and still sound smart!) *Postprandial* means "after a meal." *Reactive* relates to how your body responds to the food you eat. Some researchers have proposed the term *idiopathic postprandial syndrome* because many people who have the signs of reactive hypoglycemia don't necessarily have low blood sugar.

If you suffer from reactive hypoglycemia, your body generally reacts negatively to sugar and simple starches, because it can't handle the excess sugar load. You usually start feeling the effect about 2 to 4 hours after eating "bad" foods.

Like a Greased Pig: Easy to Define, Tough to Pin Down

Because hypoglycemia is so easy to define, you'd think that determining who has low blood sugar would be a simple matter. All you should have to do is measure the blood sugar and *voilà!* — you have inconvertible proof that someone has hypoglycemia.

Alas, it's not that cut and dried. Experts disagree on what constitutes a hypoglycemic condition. Today's standard medical practice is to consider hypoglycemic levels of blood sugar lower than 45 mg per deciliter of blood. The benchmark used to be higher, but it has shifted downward over the years, and doctors still disagree with one another in terms of finding and diagnosing the condition. For instance, some health practitioners argue *no* range of blood sugar is definitive in determining hypoglycemia; they believe instead that the speed with which the blood sugar drops is more important than how low it goes. (Chapter 5 gives you more detailed information about diagnoses and measurements.)

And that's not the only controversy surrounding hypoglycemia. These bits add to the trouble:

✔ Symptoms are nonspecific. (You can read more in Chapter 3.)

✔ Symptoms don't always correlate with blood glucose (sugar) concentrations measured during an oral glucose test. (More on this test in Chapter 5.) The rate at which the blood sugar drops is just as important, but doctors often ignore this rate.

✔ Glucose levels are rarely measured when people develop symptoms spontaneously (not easy to manage unless someone follows them around with a syringe).

✔ Hypoglycemia is a misnomer. Rather than low blood sugar, it's more a matter of the body being unable to effectively absorb certain carbohydrates. Different people react differently to ingested sugars and carbohydrates, with some having a higher tolerance level than others. Thus, the condition may be better described as *carbohydrate intolerance* or *glucose instability syndrome.*

✔ Many symptoms of hypoglycemia are caused not by the drop in blood sugar, but by the resulting glandular imbalances. For example, to counter the emergency created by the blood sugar falling too low or too rapidly, the body dumps adrenaline (epinephrine).

In the 1970s, after several books popularized hypoglycemia, many people jumped on the hypoglycemia bandwagon, and it became an over-diagnosed condition — a fad disease that most respectable healthcare practitioners strived to steer clear of. So it's understandable that many doctors are skeptical. It's also unfortunate, because they're unable to help patients who ask "If I'm so healthy, why do I feel so bad?"

Although diagnosing hypoglycemia is difficult, you can still work closely with your doctor to figure out what's causing your symptoms. This section helps you (and your doctor) get a firmer grasp on your symptoms in order to make the correct diagnosis.

Identifying key symptoms

The symptoms of hypoglycemia aren't fatal, but they can seriously detract from the quality of life. The immediate physical symptoms of low blood sugar are

- ✔ Mental confusion (brain fog)
- ✔ Inability to think rationally
- ✔ Weakness
- ✔ Shakiness

These symptoms can be alleviated by eating. The more debilitating symptoms of chronic hypoglycemia, however, are longer lasting and not immediately relieved by eating. Chapter 3 talks more about symptoms and syndromes that are often associated with hypoglycemia. We also discuss the various causes of low blood sugar in people of different age groups.

The link between food and symptoms is undeniable. Face food facts! This book can help you do that by offering alternatives to the foods you currently eat. Flip to Chapter 6 for info on the foods you can and can't safely eat as a hypoglycemic. If you have a partner and/or children, flip to Chapter 13 for help on setting up a diet lifestyle with your family.

Arriving at a diagnosis

Some people may have low blood sugar levels without hypoglycemic symptoms, while others may have symptoms of hypoglycemia, even severe ones, even though their blood sugar is within normal range. Therefore, measuring blood sugar is an unreliable way to diagnose hypoglycemia. Doctors too often ignore the rate at which the blood sugar drops, failing to recognize that some patients develop symptoms when the blood sugar falls quickly.

For these and other reasons, hypoglycemia is often dismissed as imaginary. Despite the protests of some medical organizations, many nutritionally oriented physicians, naturopaths, and other alternative practitioners assert that hypoglycemia is a real clinical entity. Instead of over-relying on glucose tests, which are often

Hit the Web for more resources

In this book we provide tons of helpful info so you can counter your hypoglycemia and not be tied down by its symptoms. However, we have only 288 pages to provide you with just the basic information. If you want more in-depth info and to keep up-to-date on what's happening in the fight against hypoglycemia and related ailments, then check out the following Web sites:

✓ **American Diabetes Association (www.diabetes.org):** This Web site provides information on diabetes, guidelines for healthy living, recipes, an e-newsletter, and an online store.

✓ **CDC Diabetes Public Health Resource (www.cdc.gov/diabetes):** Here, you can find a wide assortment of information and resources on diabetes. The Web site also has links to other good sources of information.

✓ **eMedicineHealth.com (www.emedicinehealth.com/low_blood_sugar_ hypoglycemia/article_em.htm):** This consumer health information site provides comprehensive info for first aid and emergency situations for injuries and minor medical conditions. It also provides health, medical, lifestyle, and wellness information on a variety of topics, including hypoglycemia. Physicians wrote more than 5,500 pages of content for patients and consumers.

✓ **Health Connection Radio (www.healthconnectionradio.com):** This station (WKAT 1360 AM) in South Florida has been providing information on health, wellness, and nutrition since 1996. Topics include hypoglycemia, diabetes, and alcoholism. Download the programs, hosted by Jay Foster (the director of Body Chemistry Associates and a certified clinical nutritionist), from the Web site.

✓ **Hypoglycemia Health Association of Australia (www.hypoglycemia. asn.au):** This nonprofit charitable organization provides information to its members on hypoglycemia and other nutritional disorders. It offers numerous articles, useful links to other sites, and recipes for hypoglycemics for free. The association mails newsletters, covering lectures on hypoglycemia and other related subjects, to members. Membership is $20 per year.

✓ **Hypoglycemia Homepage Holland (hypoglykemie.nl):** This Web site offers general information about hypoglycemia, as well as health tips, a newsgroup, and lists of other helpful resources.

✓ **Voice America: Health & Wellness (health.voiceamerica.com):** This Internet Talk Radio was the first to air live, online radio broadcasts. Since 1998, the station has been offering shows about a wide range of health issues discussed by physicians, alternative healthcare practitioners, writers, and others who are active in the health field. Audiences can listen to any of the station's network programs at any time through on-demand audio streaming or podcasting links. Guests featured are professionals from various walks of life, all related to health and wellness.

inaccurate, these health professionals diagnose their patients through symptoms, and successfully treat the disorder by changing their patients' diets. You can read more about these medical practitioners in Chapter 4.

The best way to diagnose the disorder is through a combination of various lab tests (which we discuss in detail in Chapter 5) and an assessment of symptoms (which we discuss in Chapter 3). In addition, you can try eliminating foods from your diet to see whether symptoms clear up. As we explain in Chapter 3, food allergies can, at times, cause hypoglycemia. The food journal we talk about in Chapter 6 can also help you determine which foods may affect you.

You should see a doctor before you do anything, especially if it's been several years since your last physical checkup.

Knowing Who's Prone

Hypoglycemia can strike anyone at any age. Unlike diabetes, not enough studies have been performed to create an accurate profile. Nevertheless, because reactive hypoglycemia can be an early sign of diabetes, it's reasonable to believe that hypoglycemics and diabetics share a genetic predisposition for metabolic disorders and similar risks for environmental triggers.

Research suggests that the following people are hypoglycemia's likeliest victims:

- ✔ Women suffering from premenstrual syndrome (PMS).
- ✔ People suffering from severe stress.
- ✔ People who are overweight (although some are underweight due to their faulty carbohydrate metabolism).
- ✔ Alcoholics. Some researchers have concluded that alcoholism is actually an unrecognized problem with body chemistry, and that all alcoholics are, in fact, hypoglycemics.

This section discusses why hypoglycemia affects certain people and briefly examines the relationship between hypoglycemia and diabetes.

Prevailing problem: The pudge!

The sugar and refined carbohydrate-laden diet that the majority of people in developed countries eat has led to a host of health problems, and hypoglycemia is one of them.

Although most medical and health organizations recommend that no more than 10 percent of total caloric intake be derived from the refined sugars added to foods, the fact is that most people in developed countries eat far more than that (possibly three times that amount), and despite recommendations, the ideal amount is zero. And what's even more alarming is that some lesser-developed Asian countries are getting a sweet tooth that rivals the richer nations! Statistics show that the consumption of sugar worldwide is increasing by 1 to 2 percent every year. Small wonder so many people have a pudge of a problem.

Like a couple of hooligans: Linking hypoglycemia and diabetes

You probably know someone who has diabetes. But you may not know that hypoglycemia and diabetes are linked. Blood sugar imbalance underlies both disorders. In the case of hypoglycemics, experts theorize that over a prolonged period of time, too much insulin (from eating sugar and simple starches) followed by a blood sugar drop results in cells losing their sensitivity to insulin. Thus, although hypoglycemia may seem to be the opposite of diabetes, it's, in fact, considered to be a pre-diabetic condition.

Both diabetics and hypoglycemics should treat their condition through dietary means. The recommended diet for diabetes and hypoglycemia is, in fact, quite similar — although low blood sugar sufferers are often advised to reduce their carbohydrate intake, at least during the early part of treatment. Chapter 3 gives more information about diabetes and hypoglycemia and how they're related. Chapter 6 gives the scoop about using your diet to your health's advantage.

Heading Toward Better Health

A paradigm shift has been taking place in recent years in most Western countries, as more people are searching for alternative practices for attaining good health — something that crisis-driven Western medicine is unable to offer. The new paradigm holds a high regard for the nutritional basis of disease. The new paradigm, with its holistic, body-mind approach to health and healing, can more fully address hypoglycemia's spectrum of problems. A *holistic* approach looks at the patient's entire lifestyle, in addition to diet, for clues to what's causing the illness.

Think of this as a journey toward greater health — a journey of transformation to a new approach to living and a greater sense of well-being. In this book, we show you how the transition into a healthy life can be smooth and not as painful as you may suspect.

The following list shows where you may be starting. If you follow the physical and food advice given in this book, you can come out on the other side looking and feeling a whole lot better.

- ✔ **Not eating right — right now:** You should be eating six small meals, or three small meals and three light snacks, per day, although you may eat more frequently if you need to when you first embark on the program. This diet is very similar to a diabetic diet and doesn't include sweets or sugars.

  If you want healthy recipes, the Internet is a great source. Plenty of good diabetes cookbooks exist as well, including the *Diabetic Cookbook For Dummies,* by Alan L. Rubin, MD, Alison G. Acerra, RD, and Chef Denise Sharf (Wiley). You can safely follow any recipes created for diabetics as long as you refrain from using artificial sweeteners.

  People are often surprisingly uninformed regarding diets and facts about hypoglycemia. Chapter 15 sets the record straight on commonly held misperceptions.

- ✔ **Overweight:** For various reasons, low blood sugar can lead to weight gain. One reason is that you may be giving in to an increased desire for sweets; Chapter 8 can help get you motivated to get moving. In addition, overeating sweets and starches overstimulates insulin production, and too much insulin causes excess storage of fat.

- ✔ **Underweight:** You may have been gorging yourself on sugars and starches in a futile attempt to gain weight. (And evoking jealousy among your friends in the process.) If so, addressing your underlying metabolism disorder can help you put on the pounds that you want and need.

- ✔ **Combating depression and mood disorders:** When Abraham Lincoln said, "People are as happy as they make up their minds to be," little knowledge existed about the basics of depression. (Ironically, evidence suggests that Lincoln himself was a generally depressed person, who never did fully "make up his mind" to be happy. Could he have suffered from hypoglycemia? Or an associated condition?) Chapter 10 talks more about depression.

- ✔ **Lacking a solid support structure:** When you have a condition that undermines your effectiveness in daily life and chips away at your confidence and self-esteem, you need a bridge. The support structure that you create for yourself is this bridge. (See? It's all up to you: Not only are you responsible for food and exercise, but finding support is all about you, too.)

A support person or group can help guide you through, especially when you're just beginning your recovery program. Chapter 12 tells you how to get the support you need. In addition, we give you plenty of online resources that can help you.

Every individual is so different that predicting a time frame of recovery is difficult, but in general, you should start to see a noticeable improvement in your health in about three months. Having an occasional bad food day won't negate your progress — but don't kid yourself. Going off your food plan for several days, not to mention weeks, will definitely impede your progress.

Chapter 2

Digesting Hypoglycemia: Your Body's Role

. . . .

In This Chapter

▶ Looking at what happens when you eat

▶ Examining potential causes of hypoglycemia

▶ Breaking the cycle: How too much sugar can lead to low blood sugar

. . . .

*B*efore you can completely understand hypoglycemia and how it affects your body, you first need to know how and why some individuals develop hypoglycemia. You needn't get a medical degree, but knowing some sweet and simple facts about sugar and how the body strives to maintain blood sugar equilibrium can most definitely help you take a proactive role in making sure that you won't have to suffer again from not having enough sugar in your bloodstream to fuel you properly.

In this chapter, we don't rhapsodize about the marvel of engineering that is the human body. We tell it like it is so that you know the hormonal basics that take place whenever you chow down. That way you can understand why diet is the cornerstone of treatment for a hypoglycemic.

Absorbing Some Physical Food

Generally, a meal provides nutrients that reach your body over a span of about four hours. However, your cells demand nutrients around the clock. (They were the first to demand 24/7 service.)

Digestion begins in your mouth — this is why your parents and other well-meaning people tell you to chew your food — and continues in your stomach. Your body has to break down the food before it can use the nutrients. The process is complex and can be a mouthful to describe in just a few words. This section breaks down the way your body digests food to help you better digest the info.

Breaking down proteins

When you bite into your favorite food (or even those lima beans you're eating because your mom taught you well), your digestive system is starting to work. The following steps show how your body breaks down proteins, beginning with that first nibble.

G'head, take a bite:

1. **Saliva comes into contact with food.**

   The salivary enzymes in the mouth partially break down some of the starch into a simple sugar called glucose. *Glucose* is the sugar in your bloodstream; it's also your body's energy source.

2. **Your body recognizes any alien proteins and breaks them down into basic amino acids.**

   Amino acids are molecular units that make up all proteins. For an example of an alien protein, think of steak. Steak is composed of protein, carbohydrates, and fat. The protein in the steak is in the form of beef protein, which doesn't do you a whole lot of good if you're a Homo sapien. (We presume you are, because you're reading this book, but if you're not — well, we've heard of stranger things!) Why? Because it has to be converted into human protein before your body can use it.

3. **Your body reconstructs some of the amino acids into human protein.**

   That protein is now available for growth, repair, and other vital physical functions.

4. **Some of the amino acids become human carbohydrates, which are converted into basic sugars: glycogen and glucose.**

   Glycogen is the sugar your body stores, mostly in the liver but also in muscle tissue. Hundreds of branches stick out from glycogen, and on each branch is glucose, which is attached to the next glucose. All are readily accessible to the glycogen-splitting enzymes.

   Your body normally converts excess glucose to glycogen or fatty acids. If you're in the fasting state, however, the *triacylglycerols* (fat stores) and amino acids produce glucose. Glycogen isn't produced. The fasting state is reached many hours after you've eaten, when the body has completely absorbed all the nutrients from the last food consumed. When the body reaches a fasting state, your body meets its energy needs by turning to nutrients that are stored in the body.

5. **The liver converts some of the excess energy into fat.**

   Excess fat is stored in the fat cells to meet long-term energy needs.

Pancreas plays its part

After your liver converts excess energy into fat, your pancreas begins its work. The *pancreas* is an organ that

✔ Manufactures *enzymes* to digest food

✔ Manufactures *bicarbonate* to neutralize stomach acid

✔ Manufactures *glucagon,* a protein hormone that stimulates the release of glucose into the blood

✔ Secretes *insulin* when alerted that you're eating carbs (Insulin is a powerful hormone that, among other things, chaperones the glucose to the body's cells, instructing the cells to take in the glucose. That's critical, because glucose is your body's fuel. For more info on insulin, check out the nearby sidebar, "What's in insulin?")

Carbohydrates are basically chains of sugar molecules. The carbs you eat are mostly chains of glucose molecules. The shorter the chain, the sweeter the taste. Some chains are longer and more complicated, having many links and even branches. Hence, short chains are known as *simple carbohydrates,* and longer ones as *complex carbohydrates.* Simple or complex, carbs are composed entirely of sugar.

If the blood delivers more glucose than the cells can take in, the liver and muscles take up the surplus.

Here's what happens to the excess glucose:

✔ The muscles hog two-thirds of the body's total store of glucose.

✔ The liver stores the other third and makes it available when the brain or other organs need to draw on the supply.

What's in insulin?

The pancreas releases insulin directly into the bloodstream to regulate the level of *glucose* (sugar) in the blood. Cells can't use glucose for energy or nourishment without insulin, which is why insulin is critical to animal and human life. Without insulin, organisms quickly die.

Insulin transports the glucose from the blood into the body's cells. It forces the liver and muscle cells to store glucose in the form of glycogen. When insulin levels are lower, the liver cells convert glycogen to glucose and excrete it into the blood.

Conversely, when insulin is released, glucose in the blood is decreased. If the level of glucose is too low, the person suffers from hypoglycemia. By definition, you have hypoglycemia if your blood sugar is too low. (Flip to Chapter 1 for a definition of hypoglycemia.)

Within the body is a constant interplay of hormones that affects the level of glucose in the blood. For instance, during periods of stress, the body releases the stress hormones epinephrine and norepinephrine (noradrenaline), which inhibit the release of insulin and increase *hepatic glycolysis,* the conversion of glycogen to glucose in the liver, thereby increasing the level of glucose available for energy.

Insulin has numerous other effects on cells, such as increased fatty acid synthesis. Insulin forces fat cells to take in blood lipids (fatty acids). The lack of insulin causes the reverse — a reduction in the uptake of blood fatty acids by cells. A reduction can mean less available energy. Other effects of insulin include increased amino acid and potassium uptake.

The following shows how the pancreas helps regulate your blood sugar level:

1. **You eat a meal, and insulin becomes the dominant hormone in your body.**

2. **Insulin is suppressed four to six hours later when glucagon shows up.**

   Glucagon shows up as your metabolism shifts gears. Glucagon suppresses insulin by releasing glucose into the blood.

   • When blood glucose levels drop too low, the pancreas releases glucagon.

   • Suppression of the insulin allows the liver to release glucose.

3. **As long as the blood glucose levels are within normal range, insulin regulates glucose metabolism.**

   If the blood glucose level dips too low, *counter-regulatory hormones* (hormones that oppose insulin's action) are released.

Insulin stores the glucose in the liver and muscle cells, and glucagon removes it from storage as needed.

Insulin gone awry

In order for your body's check-and-balance mechanism to work properly, the demand for insulin must subside at times. Assume this nasty scenario:

1. **You repeatedly chow down on snacks high in sugar and starch.**

2. **Your body has to constantly pump out insulin.**

   As a result, your body has too much insulin!

3. **The insulin receptors on the cells lose some of their sensitivity.**

4. **The pancreas secretes more insulin, hoping to get the receptors to respond.**

   Now you have way too much insulin!

5. **Insulin rounds up the glucose from the bloodstream and drives it into the cells.**

   The result is *hypoglycemia,* or low blood sugar. (Doctors who don't believe that hypoglycemia exists in so-called healthy people — in other words, nondiabetic people — would argue that hypoglycemia can't occur as just described.)

6. **The insulin receptors become desensitized, and insulin can't deliver enough glucose into the cells.**

   The result is a condition known as *insulin resistance.* See Chapter 3 for more on this condition and its link to hypoglycemia.

7. **Eventually, more sugar remains in the bloodstream.**

   The result is type 2 diabetes.

This list is an admittedly oversimplified picture and just one scenario that can cause hypoglycemia in people who are genetically susceptible. (Check out the next section for more on the causes.)

The point to remember is that when a person who's sensitive to carbs (see Chapter 3 for more) eats carbs, the blood sugar increases more rapidly than it should. This situation results in a rapid rise and fall in both insulin and blood sugar levels.

Bear in mind that carbs make up only part of the foods that directly affect blood sugar levels. Protein and fats are slowly absorbed, so the sensitive insulin apparatus is less likely to be triggered. Thus, small, regular meals consisting of protein or fats and some carbs keep the blood sugar stable, preventing sudden rises and falls in glucose.

Now you can appreciate what a complex dance the chemicals and hormones have to perform in order to keep your blood sugar level within a narrow range. The picture isn't yet complete, however. The process includes more dancers and more steps, as you see later in this chapter.

Tracing Cause and Effect

Hypoglycemia has many causes, some of which aren't related to what you eat, but this section only briefly covers them. Just remember that hypoglycemia treatment depends totally on the underlying medical illnesses. So go see your doctor first — don't diagnose yourself!

Multiple causes

Numerous factors can cause hypoglycemia, some of which are too technical for a lengthy discussion in this book. However, we do want to at least briefly tell you about the potential causes. You can check with your doctor for more scientific details.

The following are some of the causes of hypoglycemia:

- **Genes:** In some patients, low blood sugar occurs mainly because of a defect in glucose production, while in others, the problem is the result of an excessive use of glucose. Sometimes the low blood sugar level is the result of both reasons.

- **An underlying medical illness:** Although it's a matter of debate, most doctors argue that hypoglycemia doesn't occur without an underlying medical illness that's unrelated to what you eat. When a patient has no organic causes for hypoglycemia, the hormone epinephrine (adrenaline) is likely involved. It appears that insulin can stimulate epinephrine release in some sensitive people.

✔ **Profound malnutrition:** If you're severely deficient in nutrition, you're at risk for hypoglycemia because you don't have enough glucose in your blood.

✔ **Prolonged exercise:** Exercising intensely for too long without eating causes hypoglycemia because the body uses up the sugar that's stored in your liver.

✔ **Late pregnancy:** Some women may experience hypoglycemia in late pregnancy as the result of a drop in glucose production.

✔ **Severe liver deficiency:** Liver deficiencies, such as glycogen storage disease in which the body lacks enzymes responsible for forming glycogen, result in the body not being able to produce enough glucose in the blood.

✔ **Liver diseases:** These diseases include viral hepatitis and cirrhosis. Any kind of liver disease may result in a drop in blood glucose levels, because the liver stores glucose (as glycogen). The body taps into the glucose reserve in the liver for more sugar, but if the liver is diseased, it can't properly convert glycogen to glucose.

People often suffer from many of the symptoms of hypoglycemia even when their blood sugar isn't particularly low. The term *pseudo-hypoglycemia* refers to the symptoms of hypoglycemia that occur without low blood sugar.

Exhausting your adrenals

It's 11 p.m. Do you know where your adrenals are? Hopefully they're tucked away all safe and sound in bed. Seriously, if you reply that the adrenals are located above your kidneys, you're absolutely correct. The *adrenals,* which are no bigger than a walnut, rise up kind of like mushrooms from the top of each kidney and are intimately involved with normal blood sugar regulation — very important for the glycemically challenged person.

The hormones these little guys secrete influence all the major physiological processes in the body. For starters, they affect how the body uses carbs and fats, converts fats and proteins into energy, and distributes stored fat. (Remember that the next time you're in a bathing suit.)

Some researchers even believe that excessive stress is what's mostly responsible for common hypoglycemic symptoms. You may wonder how stress can have anything to do with blood sugar. The following shows you how that happens:

1. **You bounce the mortgage check, one of the kids gets the flu, and the cat barfs on your new bedspread.**

   Now that's what we call stress. (Or your average Monday.)

2. **Your adrenals work too hard and become fatigued from too much stress.**

   The adrenals react to any situation that they believe to be an emergency by secreting the hormone *adrenaline.* In the not-so-good-old-days, the fight-or-flight response was triggered when a Neanderthal man saw a rabid buffalo charging at him. More adrenaline was pumped into his bloodstream to get him ready to either fight the creature or flee. Today an emergency is more likely to be a car that cuts you off or a customer who calls you names.

3. **Cortisol levels drop lower than normal.**

   The adrenal hormone *cortisol* keeps blood sugar at adequate levels. A low level of cortisol makes maintaining normal blood sugar levels pretty tough. If your adrenals are sluggish, your liver is slow to convert glycogen to glucose. Normally, your body can convert fats, proteins, and carbs into glucose, but this process is more difficult when the adrenals are fatigued. In this situation, one of the blood sugar glitches can arise.

4. **Your liver has difficulty converting glycogen back to glucose.**

   Glycogen, or stored sugar, has to be converted into *glucose* (blood sugar) before the body can use it. When your liver has difficulty converting glycogen to glucose, less blood sugar is available, and your brain is deprived of fuel. When your brain isn't getting enough sugar, you can develop hypoglycemic symptoms, such as lightheadedness and disorientation.

Ravaging your health: The couch and the potato

In the not-so-distant past, you may have been programmed to think that carbs were not only delectable but also good for you. In more recent years, you may have gotten the impression that carbs are the root of all evil. The truth, as usual, is somewhere in between. Carbs are the most efficient fuel for the body to use, and the brain can use only sugar for its primary fuel. That may sound as if everyone should benefit from eating mega doses of carbs. But if you suffer from hypoglycemia, it may well be that your body has difficulty handling too much carbs. Even complex carbohydrates like whole grains can be problematic if your body doesn't metabolize carbs properly.

Burp. You've eaten your fill; you're stuffed to the gill. You're lying contentedly on the couch, remote in hand, relaxing after a hard day of work. Well, you may be at rest, but check this out:

1. **Your digestive tract is busier than the pizza man. It's delivering glucose to the bloodstream.**

2. **The blood carries this glucose to your liver.**

3. **The liver breaks the glucose down into small fragments and puts them together into the more permanent energy storage compound — in other words, fat.**

4. **The fat is released into the blood, carried to the body's fatty tissues, and deposited there.**

   Unlike the liver cells, which can store only about half a day's supply of glycogen, the fat cells — much to the chagrin of dieters — can store unlimited quantities of fat.

You can find out how fast carbs become glucose and enter the bloodstream by checking out the *glycemic index (GI)* of food. (See Chapter 6 for more on this topic.)

Sugar, sugar, everywhere — except where you need it

Sugar. Honey. Sweetie-pie. Terms of endearment reflect the desirability of sweet tastes. Sugar is surprisingly prevalent in dishes you may least suspect: soups, cured meats, salad dressings, and sauces, for example. One tablespoon of regular ketchup contains a teaspoon of sugar. Hoisin sauce, which you often find in Chinese cooking, has just as much sugar, if not more. A can of soda pop contains several tablespoons of sugar. Even diet foods contain large amounts of rapidly acting carbohydrates or alternative sweeteners like aspartame (which has been linked to cancer).

If you're surrounded by sugar, how can anyone possibly be suffering from low blood sugar? That's precisely the point. Because everything is so sugar-laden, keeping a steady level of blood sugar has become difficult. If someone is suffering from low blood sugar, it doesn't mean that she should eat sugar. This statement may, at first, appear to be a contradiction. The paradox is that the more sugar you eat, the less sugar you have in your blood.

Your body can easily obtain the blood sugar it needs to function through unrefined carbs, protein, and fats. The truth is that even if you eat absolutely no glucose or refined sugar, you'll still have plenty of blood sugar as long as your body is functioning properly. Chapter 6 explains why refined carbs are harmful, but unrefined carbs are okay.

Addressing Addictions: The Link to Low Blood Sugar

A sweet link may exist between various forms of addictions and low blood sugar. The connection may lie in feel-good hormones called *beta-endorphins,* which are produced in the *opioid system,* the reward pathway of the brain. Scientists are now working with the hypothesis that the presence of beta-endorphins in the reward pathway regions in the brain is key to the development of addiction to opioids like heroin. Beta-endorphins give you a feeling of euphoria, or a sense of being on top of the world.

Not surprisingly, other things can offer such addictive relationships to varying degrees. The following may help you kick your own bad habits:

- **Saying sayonara to the sauce:** The fact is, alcohol is a simple carb that's rapidly converted into sugar. It creates an addictive high that's quickly followed by a low. Hypoglycemia in alcoholics usually occurs after a several-day alcohol binge or in a malnourished state, which causes glycogen depletion in the liver and blocks glucose synthesis.

    Most treatment programs emphasize psychological factors and neglect possible biochemical deficiencies and body chemistry. Many problems attributed to an alcoholic's personality or life history may actually be caused by faulty body chemistry. If you're working toward a recovery from drinking, try addressing both your body (with dietary changes like those suggested in Chapter 6) and your mind (with support from groups like AA).

✔ **Conquering the carb crave:** Always craving the carbo rush? If so, you may be

- Getting less protein than you need

- Seeing an early warning sign that your stress level is too high (Chapter 9 shows you how to lower the boom on stress)

- Eating an out-of-balance diet

- Unconsciously using self-medication to lift your mood

✔ **Kicking caffeine in the coffeemaker:** Caffeine has an effect similar to sugar, although the results may not be so immediate. It triggers the release of stored glycogen to temporarily increase the blood sugar level. Chapter 11 offers ideas on how to kick your addiction to caffeine. Be aware that when you drink sugared, caffeinated drinks, you're essentially getting a double whammy in terms of a sugar rush! But don't be so quick to switch to diet sodas — they're not any better, because recent studies show that the artificial sweeteners used are damaging to your health. The solution? Kick your soda habit!

✔ **Knocking out nicotine:** Enough has been said about the bad effects of cigarettes and other tobacco products. But are you aware of the effect that nicotine has on blood sugar? Light up a cigarette and ping! You just boosted your blood sugar. You suddenly feel euphoric. Why? Because nicotine stimulates the adrenal glands. Unfortunately, smoking creates a desire for caffeine, sweet foods, and alcohol.

Start by adjusting your diet and taking the necessary supplements (which we describe in Chapter 7). Hypnosis, meditation, and breathing techniques may also help (see Chapter 9). If you continue to smoke, even if you follow the correct diet, you may not notice an improvement in symptoms because adrenal stimulation from the nicotine is constantly triggering the release of glucose into the blood — and the sugar spike is rapidly followed by a crash.

Chapter 3

Symptoms without a Cause

*H*aving hypoglycemia certainly isn't more fun than a barrel full of monkeys — but sometimes you may feel like monkeys are running around, keeping your mind edgy and unfocused. At times you may feel cold, anxious, or nervous; or you may be so down and depressed that you're virtually digging in the ditches. (If that's the case, check out Chapter 10.) Then, before you know it, your heart is racing so fast that you'd think you were running from a herd of elephants. Meanwhile, you're experiencing memory loss; it's getting so that you can't remember what you've forgotten.

If you often experience these symptoms, you may have chronic hypoglycemia. Or not. Determining whether you have this disorder can be downright confusing, because the symptoms mimic so many other illnesses. This chapter clarifies the muddy waters. (For information about getting a proper medical diagnosis from a doctor, turn to Chapter 5.) This chapter also makes clear the connection between diabetes and hypoglycemia.

Jumping on Stage: No, You're Not Faking It

Nothing's clear cut about hypoglycemia. Why would its stages be any different? Generally speaking, doctors can detect two basic stages. Each stage can last anywhere from weeks to years, depending on the individual and the underlying cause. In fact, though, these stages aren't so clear-cut. They may come and go, and they can possibly overlap.

✔ **Stage 1:** Depression, fatigue, lethargy, poor concentration, and memory loss

✔ **Stage 2:** Agitation, fast heartbeat, cold and clammy hands, and possibly full-blown panic attacks

That's the fun part. The not-so-fun part is that most people are going to label you a hypochondriac. As far as they're concerned, the problem's all in your mind. And no wonder; hypoglycemia has just too many darn symptoms. (For more information on talking about the disorder with those you know and love, check out Chapters 13 and 14.) When confronted with the long list of nonspecific complaints that hypoglycemics generally present, many doctors may be tempted to dismiss it as hogwash. (That's the medical term for "I'd rather scrub Porky Pig in a tub than deal with this.") Don't let the doctor's diagnosis deter you. Find a doctor or healthcare practitioner who truly understands hypoglycemia. (See Chapter 4.)

If you suspect that you may have hypoglycemia, get a proper checkup to rule out other causes for your symptoms. The kind of chronic hypoglycemia we talk about in this book may be disabling, but it's not fatal. If something else is causing your low blood sugar, you can end up harming yourself by not getting proper treatment. (See "Unmasking Hypoglycemia's Hidden Faces" later in this chapter for various causes of hypoglycemia.)

Eying the Physical Symptoms

If you're like most people with hypoglycemia, you wake up feeling tired and exhausted, and your body may feel achy. You may not feel good in the morning, but you usually feel much better in the evening. (Generally, people have higher levels of blood sugar in the evening.)

The long and short of it is that a long list of physical symptoms is classically attributed to hypoglycemia. When checking out this list, look for a group of symptoms that *persist over time*.

Here are just some of the symptoms associated with hypoglycemia:

✔ Accident prone

✔ Aching eye sockets

✔ Backache and muscle pain

✔ Bad breath

✔ Hot flashes

✔ Chronic indigestion

✔ Internal trembling

✔ Itching, crawling skin sensations

- ✔ Blurred vision
- ✔ Chatterbox (talking a lot)
- ✔ Chronically cold hands and feet
- ✔ Convulsions
- ✔ Dizziness
- ✔ Drowsiness
- ✔ Fainting or blackouts
- ✔ Family history of diabetes or low blood sugar
- ✔ Fatigue or exhaustion
- ✔ Headaches
- ✔ Heart palpitations

- ✔ Joint pain
- ✔ Muscular twitching or cramps
- ✔ Numbness
- ✔ Obesity
- ✔ Premenstrual symptoms
- ✔ Ringing in ears
- ✔ Sensitivity to light and noise
- ✔ Excessive sighing and yawning
- ✔ Difficulty sleeping
- ✔ Excessive sweating

 How many of these symptoms do you have? If you've experienced a few or more, congratulations: It proves that you're not the living dead. Everyone is bound to have some of these symptoms at some time. If you have a few, especially of short duration, don't worry. Even if you experience the symptoms fairly regularly, other conditions may be causing them. For instance, hot flashes may be due to the fact that you're a female of a certain age. And as for itching and crawling sensations on the skin — don't look now, but there's a spider on your arm. Not everything under the sun can be blamed on low blood sugar.

 Some symptoms can indicate a serious problem. See a doctor immediately if you experience dizziness, numbness, fainting, or convulsions.

Identifying the Emotional Symptoms

People tend to behave in a bizarre manner when their tanks are running on empty (or when their blood glucose is low). You can't run without fuel, and you accept that. So how can you expect your brain to work without the proper fuel — and in the case of that hefty gray matter (which we describe further in Chapter 2), the fuel of choice is glucose. Starve your poor brain and you may have bizarre behavioral symptoms that can look like dementia, paranoia, or even schizophrenia.

PMS? Yes!

Premenstrual syndrome (PMS) is often associated with increased appetite, a craving for sweets, headaches, fatigue, and heart palpitations — in fact, all the symptoms of hypoglycemia. It's no wonder. Glucose tolerance tests given to premenstrual subjects showed excess insulin in response to sugar consumption. It appears that women who suffer from PMS have incidents of hypoglycemia that correlate with their menstrual cycles.

If you're a woman who has experienced PMS, you know that you often crave something sweet and simple, such as sugar and flour, just before your period. It's the low blood sugar talking. Most women who devour sugar and simple starches experience stress, anxiety, and moodiness just before their periods — 80 to 90 percent of the sugar eaters, according to some research. The problem is easily rectified by changing your diet. Try to follow the diet recommended for hypoglycemics (see Chapter 6), especially when you feel an attack of PMS coming on.

Here's an extensive (but by no means complete) list of mental symptoms that can be induced by hypoglycemia:

- Antisocial behavior
- Circular thinking
- Constant worrying
- Difficulty in concentration
- Emotional fragility
- Exhaustion
- Feeling on edge
- Feelings of going mad or insane
- Feelings of inadequacy
- Forgetfulness
- Indecisiveness
- Irritability

- Lack of sex drive
- Low tolerance for stress
- Mental confusion (brain fog)
- Moodiness
- Negative thoughts and attitudes
- Nervousness
- Night terrors, nightmares
- Phobias
- Restlessness
- Suicidal thoughts or tendencies
- Temper tantrums

Of course, everyone experiences some of these emotional states at some time or other. (If you're convinced that you don't, ask your loved ones: They'll tell you otherwise!) What you should look out for are regular and extended bouts with these symptoms. By following the dietary guidelines and keeping a food journal like the one we discuss in Chapter 6, you can make correlations to the foods, moods, and behaviors that affect you. If you suffer from nightmares, night sweats, or sleeplessness, check out the nearby sidebar, "Snacking before bed: It's a go."

Seek professional help immediately if you experience suicidal thoughts/tendencies or mental confusion.

Unmasking Hypoglycemia's Hidden Faces

It may seem as though hypoglycemia is blamed for just about every condition under the sun. Maybe the stock market dive will eventually be attributed to low blood sugar. (The idea isn't as far-fetched as you may think. During the "bubble economy," some people speculated that the skyrocketing economy was caused in part by investors feeling terribly optimistic after taking Prozac.)

What's confounding about hypoglycemia is that practically every one of its symptoms can be caused by other *pathological conditions* — diseases and illnesses that have other causes. If you're suffering from symptoms that are suggestive of hypoglycemia, one of the following may be true:

Snacking before bed: It's a go

Insulin regulation plays a role in your sleeping habits. If you're prone to low blood sugar, you may often have nightmares, night sweats, and sleeplessness. When you go without eating for many hours during the night, your blood glucose can plunge. This plunge in blood glucose levels dropkicks your adrenals into gear. Your adrenals then release adrenaline as a secondary energy source. Because adrenaline is a stimulatory hormone, it keeps you from having a sound, peaceful sleep.

To avoid the effects of adrenaline, have a light snack just before going to bed. Yogurt and cottage cheese are good choices. If you have a weight problem, make sure that the snack isn't something that's high in calories. Remember, you don't need to eat a lot — and avoid foods, such as simple starches, that will cause your body to produce too much insulin.

✔ Hypoglycemia may be the hidden cause. In other words, you have these symptoms because you have hypoglycemia.

✔ The hypoglycemic symptom may indicate a different illness. The symptoms you have are the result of a different condition, not hypoglycemia.

✔ Hypoglycemia is paired with another condition. You have two conditions, one of which is hypoglycemia. In these cases, hypoglycemia may lead to the other condition, or the other condition may lead to hypoglycemia. Or, in some cases, you may be suffering from more than one syndrome in addition to hypoglycemia. Sorting everything becomes terribly difficult.

You can safely follow virtually the same, basic hypoglycemic diet — with perhaps some modifications based on individual needs and circumstances — regardless of whether you suffer from one or more of the other syndromes we discuss in the following sections. But if you see little or no improvement in your condition after several months of following a hypoglycemic diet (see Chapter 6), you may need to get more specific treatment for your other conditions, including fine-tuning your diet. In this case, follow the guidance of an experienced health practitioner.

You don't have to worry about harming yourself by following a hypoglycemic diet. It's a safe and sound way of eating. Unlike fad diets, the hypoglycemic diet can only improve your health, not hurt it.

Untangling what's caused by what can be quite tricky, because the symptoms can overlap. For example, persistent fatigue, mood disorders, and brain dysfunctions, such as impaired memory and concentration — all hallmarks of hypoglycemia — are also symptoms of hypothyroidism and chronic fatigue syndrome. We can't cover every single condition related to hypoglycemia, but the following sections discuss a few of the major ones.

Reactions to food

If your doctor mentions food reactions, she's not talking about your food likes and dislikes. She's referring to allergies, tolerances, or sensitivities to certain foods. When you're allergic or sensitive to a food, eating it provokes a reaction, such as a rash or hives.

Even if you're not truly allergic to a substance, your body may still react to it. For instance, have you ever eaten at a Chinese restaurant and hours later experienced headaches, nausea, dizziness, and other uncomfortable symptoms? It could be a reaction to monosodium glutamate (MSG), which is used in many Chinese dishes.

Food allergy

A *food allergy* is an adverse reaction of your body's immune system to a food. A true allergy, as defined by medicine, shows a certain level of immune cells or antibodies on blood tests. An allergic response is usually immediate. The reaction can range from mild to serious, and is sometimes even life-threatening.

People are most often allergic to milk, eggs, peanuts, tree nuts, soy, wheat, fish, and shellfish. Alternative practitioners of integrative medicine recognize a broader definition of allergies that includes delayed reaction to foods.

Food intolerance

A *food intolerance* is an inability to properly digest various foods due to lack of certain enzymes in your body. The best known example is lactose intolerance. A lactose intolerant person can't drink milk without getting an unpleasant reaction.

Food sensitivity

Food sensitivity is a catch-all term that's often used to cover any adverse food reactions. You can be sensitive to foods without suffering from an allergy or a food intolerance. Food sensitivities can show up as physical, mental, or emotional symptoms. Reactions are usually delayed; they may occur days or even weeks after you eat the offending food. Symptoms, such as sinus congestion, asthma, and headaches, may linger and recur.

Some researchers suspect that food sensitivities may be implicated in hypoglycemia — as well as a host of other conditions, including depression, chronic fatigue syndrome, candidiasis, fibromyalgia, rheumatoid arthritis, and so forth.

Food sensitivities may affect the brain and the central nervous system, resulting in various syndromes. For example, chronic food intolerances may lead to anxiety, irritability, and hyperactivity in both adults and children. Sensitivities aren't restricted to just food. If you're susceptible to food sensitivities, you may experience toxic reactions to chemicals and pollutants in the environment as well. These irritants include pesticides, carpeting, bleach, food colorings, and food additives, to name just a few.

Western, allopathic doctors may scoff at the notion that food reactions could be responsible for such a wide array of conditions. But many sufferers assert that they've found relief from symptoms by eliminating offending foods or substances.

Coping with food reactions

If you suspect that you may be reacting adversely to certain foods, then by all means keep a food journal. Chapter 6 tells you how. After keeping a record for two to three weeks, review your journal. Do you detect a pattern? Do you find a correlation between your symptoms and certain foods? You may find that you're sensitive to foods that you often crave or eat frequently (if you commonly crave bread or pasta, check out the nearby sidebar "Glutton for gluten"). Try eliminating the suspected foods for at least five days to see whether your symptoms clear.

Not sure where to start? Go on an elimination diet by trying the following for two weeks:

✔ Remove the most common offenders — milk, eggs, peanuts, tree nuts, soy, wheat, fish, and shellfish.

✔ Remove corn and citrus foods; some people are bothered by these foods.

✔ Consume only vegetables and boiled or broiled meat.

✔ Consume fresh fruits if your system can handle them.

✔ Drink plenty of water.

✔ Continue keeping your food journal.

At the end of the trial, add one food at a time back into your diet. Eat this food for four days. Be sure to note in your food journal any reactions to the food (check out Chapter 6 for more on keeping a journal). Repeat the process with each food that you eliminated. When symptoms return after reintroducing a certain food, then you've likely identified a culprit.

After you identify offending foods, stop consuming them. Most people start feeling better quite rapidly. You may find that after a long period of abstaining from a particular food, you can eat it with no problem. The method we describe here requires time, planning, and effort, but it also has benefits; for example, this method

✔ Is regarded as one of the best ways of ferreting out food intolerances

✔ Costs much less than getting tests for food sensitivities, which can be quite expensive and not necessarily any more accurate

✔ Helps you become better acquainted with your body's unique needs

If at any time you start to experience severe reactions, such as vomiting, wheezing, or a swollen throat, stop self-testing and consult an allergist at once.

Overlapping syndromes

Teasing out different symptoms is rather like trying to untangle a ball of yarn. A lot of syndromes overlap. This situation is particularly true of fibromyalgia, candidiasis, and chronic fatigue syndrome, which share so many symptoms.

Fibromyalgia

Fibromyalgia syndrome (FMS) is a disorder that affects mostly women. The cause is still unknown. Patients typically suffer from

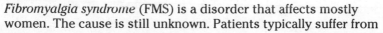

Glutton for gluten

Do you crave breads, pasta, and other wheat-based products? If so, you may have a gluten sensitivity or allergy. *Gluten* is the protein that's in wheat, rye, barley, and perhaps oats as well. (Oats don't contain gluten, but because they're handled by the same mills that process wheat, barley, and rye, they may be contaminated with gluten. So avoid oats unless you buy them from companies that provide non-contaminated oats.) Gluten may be the most common food intolerance. Considering that you can find it in such all-time favorite foods as bread, pasta, cakes, cookies, and pizza crust, you can see that gluten sensitivity can be a serious problem.

This info may sound paradoxical, but people with food intolerances may actually crave the very food that their body is unable to handle. The more you crave it, the more you eat it, and the more havoc it plays in your system.

A genetic disorder called celiac disease, which results in damage to the intestine, may be at the root of gluten intolerance in some people. Celiac disease can provoke a complex range of different reactions, not all of them digestive issues like gas, diarrhea, constipation, or abdominal pain. Symptoms may also include impaired brain function, depression, joint pain, and fatigue. The disease can't be cured, but it can be managed by simply avoiding gluten.

Although only a small minority of people is diagnosed with this disease, suffering from some degree of gluten sensitivity without actually having celiac disease is possible. If you're one of these people, you can dramatically improve your health by eliminating all gluten from your diet. As an added bonus, the gluten-free diet is highly compatible with the hypoglycemic diet.

For more info, check out *Living Gluten-Free For Dummies,* by Dana Korn (Wiley).

fatigue, irritability, nervousness, depression, anxiety, sleep disorder, and cognitive and memory impairment. Fibromyalgia patients can also have a blood sugar imbalance that exacerbates their condition.

How can you tell FMS from hypoglycemia? Through your pain. Although hypoglycemia can cause some muscle aches and joint pain, FMS patients generally ache all over: They experience pain in the muscles, ligaments, and tendons. They have specific spots on the body (called *tender points*) that hurt when pressed with enough pressure to whiten the thumbnail. They may also have genitourinary (cystitis, vaginal spasms, and so on) and gastrointestinal complaints (bloating, gas, and constipation alternating with diarrhea). Interested in knowing more? Check out *Fibromyalgia For Dummies,* by Roland Staud, MD, and Christine Adamec (Wiley).

Candidiasis

Your immune system and the presence of beneficial bacteria in your gut usually inhibit the overgrowth of *candida albican,* a fungi normally found in the body, particularly in the mouth, vagina, and intestinal tract.

If you're stressed, have an infection, experience a nutritional imbalance, or regularly use birth control pills, cortisone, or antibiotics over a long period of time, candida can proliferate and change to a fungoid form. Some people believe that this fungoid form can damage the intestinal lining and produce a wide range of symptoms (many of which are the same as the symptoms caused by hypoglycemia).

Candidiasis and hypoglycemia go hand in hand; if you have one of these two conditions, you just may have the other, too. Why? Because many people afflicted with hypoglycemia are also prone to having a sweet-tooth or a carb-craving that contributes to their blood sugar problems. (Okay, many of them are downright sugar addicts!) And sweets and simple carbs — which turn into sugar in the gut — spread yeast infections by feeding the candida!

Nothing proves that candidiasis exists as a disease state, and many doctors, including Dr. Chow (this book's co-author), are extremely careful about making a diagnosis of candidiasis. Be wary of practitioners who readily blame candidiasis for all kinds of health problems. Take a careful medical history and keep a meticulously accurate food journal. (See Chapter 6 for information on how to keep your own food journal.)

You may have reason to suspect candidiasis if you have a few of the following conditions:

✔ Recurrent yeast infections

✔ Vaginal burning, itching, or discharge that proves resistant to treatment

✔ History of cortisone or antibiotic therapy

✔ History of thrush or chronic cystitis

✔ Symptoms of hypoglycemia that are resistant to treatment

Going on a hypoglycemic diet can be very helpful if you think that you have candidiasis. In addition, avoid foods that contain yeast or are made with a fermentation process, including mature cheeses, vinegar, mushrooms, yogurt, sauerkraut, soy sauce, honey, oranges, and pickles.

Chronic fatigue syndrome

To make matters even more complex, *chronic fatigue syndrome* (CFS) can coexist with fibromyalgia (and hypoglycemia can coexist quite merrily with both these syndromes). In fact, CFS is quite similar to fibromyalgia.

A key CFS symptom is severe, unexplained fatigue that's not relieved by rest and that lasts for at least six or more consecutive months. Other symptoms may include cognitive problems (lack of concentration, memory loss), sore throat without signs of infection, unrestful sleep, muscle pain, and headaches.

Haggling with hypothyroidism

Are you overweight? Are you tired, irritable, and constipated? Do you have headaches or a bad case of premenstrual syndrome? Do you seem to be allergic to everything, and, for crying out loud, are you losing your hair?

If you're experiencing these symptoms, you may very well have *hypothyroidism,* a condition where your thyroid gland doesn't produce enough of the hormone that regulates your metabolism. When you have too little thyroid hormone, you may experience depression, chronic fatigue, circulatory problems, compulsive overeating, and irritable bowel syndrome (whose symptoms include gas with alternating constipation and diarrhea).

According to some practitioners, hypothyroidism is eight times more common in women than in men, and it's also an associated condition of hypoglycemia. In other words, low blood sugar can be caused by hypothyroidism, in which case you need to get your thyroid taken care of as soon as possible. You should change your diet, as well. Eating wholesome, nourishing foods is always a good idea.

Joining the hypo bandwagon: Hypoadrenalism

The adrenal glands are two very small glands above each kidney. Although these glands are small, they're very important, because they produce various hormones. *Hypoadrenalism (hypoadrenia),* or adrenal insufficiency, occurs when your adrenal glands become depleted, causing a decrease in the output of adrenal hormones, including cortisol, which is released in response to stress. Cortisol increases blood pressure and blood sugar levels.

The extreme form of this condition, known as *Addison's disease,* can be life threatening if untreated. Fortunately it's quite rare, but if you do have it, you're in good company. President John Kennedy had adrenal insufficiency most of his life.

Less severe forms of low adrenal function (also called adrenal fatigue) can cause weight gain, fatigue, sleep disturbances, depression, and panic attacks. And yes, these symptoms do sound disturbingly similar to the hypoglycemic symptoms. Modern medicine (mainstream Western medical practice) doesn't recognize the low-end, non-Addison's adrenal fatigue as a distinct syndrome. But many healthcare practitioners claim to have seen many patients who suffer from diminished activity of the adrenal glands. And — here's the link to hypoglycemia — they believe that sluggish adrenal function can lead to low blood sugar.

Like sufferers of hypoglycemia, individuals whose adrenals are exhausted often crave caffeine or carbs for a quick pick-me-up. You may be suffering from either or both hypoglycemia and adrenal fatigue. You can purchase salivary cortisol tests online to help you see whether you have impaired adrenal function. You can take the test at home and get the results from a lab. However, because cortisol levels vary with the time of day, you'll get more accurate readings if you take four separate tests at different times.

In most cases, following the recommended dietary and lifestyle changes we describe in this book can help with adrenal fatigue. If those changes don't help, go to a nutritionally oriented medical doctor or naturopath. (Chapter 5 deals with lab tests, and Chapter 4 talks about alternative health practitioners.)

Because prolonged stress can lead to adrenal fatigue and exhaustion, managing stress is critical to your health and well-being. (Chapter 9 gives you tips on stress-busting.) Be sure to get plenty of rest and exercise. And do something fun for yourself for 15 minutes or more every day.

Hypoglycemia and Diabetes — Flip Sides of the Same Coin?

If you remember one thing from this book, make sure it's this: Insulin plays a critical role in your metabolism, which is directly related to your health, energy, and well-being. Hormones such as insulin, even a tiny amount, have incredibly powerful effects on the body. (For more on insulin, flip to Chapter 2.)

Both diabetics and hypoglycemics have a glitch in their insulin functioning. Because insulin sweeps away blood sugar, excess insulin can lead to a drop in blood sugar. Sugars and simple starches trigger a greater insulin response than other foods, which is one reason why hypoglycemics are advised to stay away from them.

This section delves deeper into the connection between diabetes and hypoglycemia so you can better understand the severity if you suspect you have hypoglycemia.

Looking at the syndrome flowchart

Although it's still a point of discussion, many researchers believe that hypoglycemia can be seen as a pre-diabetic form of glucose intolerance, which can eventually develop into full-blown diabetes in people who are genetically predisposed to diabetes. In other words, diabetes and hypoglycemia may fall on the continuum of the same degenerative disease (see Figure 3-1).

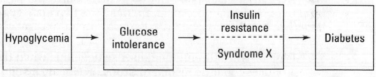

Figure 3-1: The possible progression of syndromes.

Hypoglycemia starts with impaired glucose tolerance and then develops into insulin resistance. People with insulin resistance often also suffer from heart risk factors, such as elevated blood pressure, low HDL cholesterol (the "good" kind), and abdominal obesity. Some researchers have begun calling a collection of these features *Syndrome X*. Bear in mind that there's no clear-cut point where one syndrome ends and the next one begins. If left untreated, hypoglycemia may progress into other metabolic conditions that culminate in type 2 diabetes.

✔ **Impaired glucose tolerance:** This is a pre-diabetic condition in which the body is no longer able to use glucose well. The cells are beginning to lose their sensitivity to insulin, and they don't readily respond when insulin tries to deliver glucose to them, so the body produces more insulin.

✔ **Insulin resistance:** Even as the body is producing more insulin, the cells are losing their sensitivity to insulin. The task of insulin is to deliver blood sugar to cells but, in this stage, blood sugar remains in the bloodstream even when the cells stop responding. (Check out the nearby sidebar, "Insulin resistance and the miracle 'cure'" for more info.)

✔ **Syndrome X:** Sounds like a mystery novel, doesn't it? Although you're not dealing with a murder mystery here, Syndrome X can indeed be deadly. This pre-diabetic condition is also known as *insulin resistance syndrome* or *metabolic cardiovascular risk syndrome* (MCVS). The underlying problem in people with Syndrome X is that their body is insensitive to insulin. (Think of it as insulin resistance with a few other "baddies" thrown in.) Other characteristics of Syndrome X include elevated blood cholesterol and *triglycerides* (fatty acids that normally circulate in the blood) and high blood pressure.

✔ **Diabetes (type 2):** This condition is a chronic syndrome of impaired fat, carbohydrate, and protein metabolism due to insufficient secretion of insulin or to insulin resistance. Blood sugar level remains elevated after fasting.

Identifying the types of diabetes

Some researchers suspect that 60 percent of people who suffer from hypoglycemia become diabetics. The two main types of diabetes are

✔ **Type 1:** This autoimmune disease develops when the pancreas produces too little insulin or stops producing insulin altogether. The disease may also be caused by a viral infection. Type 1 diabetes was previously known as *juvenile diabetes* because it's usually diagnosed in children and young adults.

✔ **Type 2:** This type of diabetes and hypoglycemia are like mirror images of each other. You may think of diabetes and hypoglycemia as part of the continuum of a progressive disease, with hypoglycemia at one end and diabetes at the other. Many practitioners believe that hypoglycemia can develop into type 2 diabetes, although this is a matter of debate. What most people do agree on is that a poor diet is the contributing factor — if not *the* cause — in both diabetes and hypoglycemia. Both are chronic degenerative diseases that respond to dietary and lifestyle changes.

If you have a brother or sister with type 2 diabetes, you have about a 40 percent chance of getting the illness. If you have one parent with the disease, you have a 10 percent chance of getting it. Although genetic inheritance plays a part in the development of type 2 diabetes, diet and lifestyle can help prevent it. Excess weight — obesity is a major contributing factor to type 2 diabetes — and lack of exercise can trigger diabetes. Switching to a healthy diet and working out regularly can considerably reduce your risk factor.

If you're a low blood sugar sufferer, check into your family's medical history. When you look at the family medical history of hypoglycemics, you often find that they have close family members with either hypoglycemia or type 2 diabetes. For more info about diabetes, check out *Diabetes For Dummies,* by Alan L. Rubin, MD (Wiley). The book gives a thorough explanation of both types.

Insulin resistance and the miracle "cure"

What is insulin resistance? Your body's cells stop responding to insulin, leading to excess sugar remaining in the blood, which is a symptom of diabetes. Chronic hypoglycemia can lead to insulin resistance. (Flip to "Looking at the Syndrome flowchart" earlier in this chapter.) Recent studies suggest that insulin resistance is an even greater risk factor for heart attack than either HDL cholesterol or triglycerides levels.

If you happen to be one of the growing number of people with insulin resistance, don't despair. You can still beat the odds of developing diabetes with something as simple and ordinary as regular exercise.

Scientists know that exercise improves insulin resistance and reduces the risk of adult-onset type 2 diabetes. Apparently, exercise is effective in younger people as well. A recent study focusing on 22 overweight teens found that after 16 weeks of twice-weekly resistance training, insulin sensitivity significantly increased. During the study, the adolescents' body composition changed (body fat percentage decreased and muscle mass increased), but even after adjusting for those changes in body composition, insulin sensitivity improved considerably. The study surveyed 22 Latino youths. According to the American Diabetes Association, Latinos are 17 times more likely to be diabetic than white adolescents.

Nailing Down Hypoglycemia: Symptoms throughout the Ages

No matter how old (or young) a person is, hypoglycemia can cause irritating and even debilitating symptoms, but it can affect people at different ages in different ways. Although the normal range of blood sugar levels varies with age, some people exhibit symptoms even with blood sugar levels well within the normal range. Others remain free of symptoms even when the blood sugar drops below that normal range. (Turn to Chapter 1 for more about the difficulties of accurately identifying hypoglycemia.)

Don't start worrying and don't become preoccupied about what might go wrong. Living a happy and healthy life is possible at any age if you stick to a healthy diet (see Chapter 6) and a sensible exercise program (see Chapter 8). A regular weight-bearing exercise is particularly beneficial in regulating blood sugar.

The bottom line: Hypoglycemia can occur at any age. In this section, we look at how this condition affects people at different stages in their lives.

Hypoglycemia and newborns

Being able to tell when babies and toddlers are suffering from hypoglycemia is difficult. Possible symptoms include jitteriness, poor feeding, lethargy, and low body temperature.

A baby's blood sugar may be low immediately after delivery if the mother was diabetic during pregnancy. The fetal pancreas releases more insulin to balance Mom's excess blood sugar. Such a baby is referred to as an IDM (infant of diabetic mother). Other causes for hypoglycemia in newborn children include nutritional deficiency during pregnancy; prolonged fasting, if something keeps the baby from feeding properly; liver disease in the newborn; premature birth; and unusually low birth weight.

Hypoglycemia is very common in association with certain *congenital* (since birth) hereditary disorders of metabolism. Babies in families with a history of genetically based metabolic disorders need appropriate medical tests to screen for possible problems.

Hypoglycemia and children

Children may suffer from hypoglycemia if they have diarrhea, growth hormone deficiency, or some congenital disorder resulting in the production of excess insulin. If a child suddenly shows symptoms like those of hypoglycemia, make sure that she hasn't accidentally swallowed something potentially toxic, such as medication meant for someone else.

Older children and teenagers may experience episodes of hypoglycemia if they skip meals or eat sugar-laden, high-carbohydrate junk foods. As in adults, poor eating habits can lead to feelings of shakiness, fatigue, and other problems.

 Make sure your kids aren't grabbing just donuts or candy bars — which can lead to a blood sugar crash — for breakfast. Encourage them to follow the diet outlined in Chapter 6 as much as possible.

Hypoglycemia and pregnant women

Even if you never had hypoglycemia before you got pregnant, if you start experiencing fatigue, weakness, dizziness, nausea, and other signs and symptoms of hypoglycemia, you may well be suffering from it. It's most likely a temporary bout of hypoglycemia that clears up after pregnancy, but be sure to let your doctor know.

Follow a healthy diet and you'll give birth to a healthy baby. Of course, it's not quite that simple. But you'll certainly improve the odds of a healthy birth by sticking to a healthy diet. If your diet hasn't been quite so healthy, pregnancy may be a great motivation for improvement. A proper diet is especially important during this period because the changing hormone levels during pregnancy may make you prone to blood sugar imbalance, either hypoglycemia or diabetes. Appropriate exercise is also beneficial to pregnant women, but if you're prone to low blood sugar, make sure you eat a small pre-exercise snack and another snack right after working out.

 Be extra careful in keeping your blood sugar balanced. Consult your gynecologist about how best to handle a hypoglycemic or diabetic sugar imbalance during your pregnancy.

Hypoglycemia and menopausal women

We hate to be the bearer of bad news. But the truth is, in some cases, hypoglycemia can aggravate menopausal symptoms, and vice versa. Symptoms such as depression, headaches, dizziness, and heart palpitations may become more pronounced if you're a hypoglycemic undergoing menopause. Imagine adding hypoglycemic symptoms to the normal challenges of fluctuating hormone levels!

Sticking to your hypoglycemic diet is the key to remaining healthy. After you reach middle age, you may find that you have to be even more rigorous with your diet. Alcohol and sweets, always a no-no for hypoglycemics, may cause more problems for you as your body changes with age.

Hypoglycemia and older people

As you age, the risk of hypoglycemia may increase. Because older people often take a number of different medications, they sometimes suffer from hypoglycemia brought on by complex drug interactions. Other possible causes are hormone-related, such as adrenal insufficiency (adrenal glands not producing enough cortisol in response to stress) or hypopituitarism (pituitary gland not producing normal amounts of hormones).

A patient with type 2 diabetes is always at greater risk of hypoglycemia due to the insulin or other medication he takes to lower his blood sugar. This risk may be heightened as the diabetic gets older. If a diabetic who takes insulin also has chronic renal (kidney) failure, the risk of hypoglycemia increases considerably.

If you're a senior citizen, or if you're taking care of one, know that an older person's awareness of hypoglycemia's tell-tale signs may be diminished. Therefore, even if the senior citizen doesn't think he has hypoglycemia, if he undergoes a sudden or profound change of mental state, or if he becomes agitated without apparent cause, make sure to screen for hypoglycemia in addition to any other screening your physician recommends. His cognitive difficulties may be caused by hypoglycemia and not senility.

Because older people sometimes have difficulty absorbing nutrients properly, vitamins and other dietary supplements may benefit them greatly. (Flip to Chapter 7 for information on herbs, vitamins, and other kinds of supplements.) Always consult your healthcare provider to see what may work best for you.

Part II

Diagnosing and Treating Your Hypoglycemia

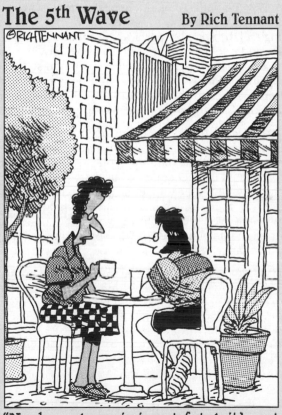

The 5th Wave   By Rich Tennant

"No, hypoglycemia is not fatal, it's not contagious, and it doesn't mean you'll always get half my desserts."

In this part . . .

Perhaps a chance remark or something you read gave you some cause to suspect that you or your loved one may be hypoglycemic. This part provides essential info to help you find a doctor who understands your symptoms and determine whether you really do suffer from hypoglycemia (or some other related condition). We describe and cover the underlying biochemistry behind hypoglycemia, as well as how to get tested. We help you sort through all the complexities and permutations of this syndrome and rule out other possible causes for what's ailing you. Because hypoglycemia means low blood sugar, we talk about sugar a lot: what it is, how your body metabolizes it, and what it does to your health. Ah, such a sweet subject, sugar. But it's a bittersweet one, as this part tells you.

We also discuss the role of nutrition in health, particularly the great significance it has for the hypoglycemic person. You discover that the only way you can recover from hypoglycemia is by changing your diet. Nothing else you do can have the same impact on your health. It doesn't matter how many flower essences you inhale, herbs or supplements you quaff, mantras you chant, or acupuncture treatments you receive: The bottom line is that you have to change your diet.

After you make the change, you may want to supplement your diet with vitamins, herbs, and supplements. This part has a chapter complete with different supplements that may help relieve some of your symptoms.

Chapter 4

Matching Up with the Right Doc

*Y*ou'd probably rather recline on a couch than trying to recline in a clinic waiting room, right? But hey, everyone has to do it sooner or later. Rather than jump to conclusions about your health, you owe it to yourself to get a thorough physical check-up to make sure that you get a proper diagnosis of your hypoglycemia symptoms. And you need to make sure that your low blood sugar isn't due to other causes or something totally unrelated. Only when you've ruled out other illnesses can you begin the proper treatment. The danger of self-diagnosis is that you may be treating yourself for a problem that doesn't even exist, while the real disease goes untreated.

This chapter discusses the importance of visiting a doctor on a regular basis to monitor your hypoglycemia and how you can find the right doctor for you. If you want to see a specialist, this chapter helps you, and if you're interested in alternative medicines, this chapter provides helpful info to manage your hypoglycemia.

Why Seeing a Doc on a Regular Basis Is Important

When dealing with your health, you have to be proactive and take charge. If you're too weak, fatigued, depressed, or whatever to muster up the energy and clarity of mind, assign someone you trust to take care of things for you. If no family member or friend can help, consider paying a professional, or perhaps a therapist or a life coach. Hiring a pro obviously costs more, but the expenses are only temporary. And you'll feel better.

After all is said and done, treating hypoglycemia is surprisingly simple and low-tech. Avoid refined sugars and starches, eat high-quality protein and whole, natural foods, and exercise regularly. Get a good belly laugh every day. Most of your treatment plan starts with your doctor, who can help you lead a healthier lifestyle and monitor your progress.

You may avoid the doctor's office because you're afraid of needles. We confess that *some* minor discomfort *may* be involved, depending on what tests your doctor administers, but standard physicals are pretty much pain-free. And we promise you that the experience is much less traumatic than that time you were abducted by space aliens. The medical staff is much more human, for one thing; they're basically nice folks who want you to feel comfortable and relaxed.

 Keeping on top of your health, with the help of your primary care physician (PCP), is extremely important. You can identify problems — and potential problems — earlier and nip them in the bud. Don't wait until you're in dire need of medical attention before you see a doctor; preventing problems is often easier than treating them.

Okay, okay — the lecture's over. Now go make an appointment with a doctor. Do you know who you should see? Maybe you're not sure. In that case, read on; this chapter helps you determine who you should hire (and maybe fire) and lets you know what to expect when you get a physical. If you'd rather see an alternative health practitioner, we have suggestions for finding one of those, too.

Paging Dr. Perfection

You may have to put forth some effort when trying to find a good doctor for treating your symptoms of hypoglycemia. Aside from being competent and having the proper credentials, your doctor should be caring and compassionate.

We advocate finding a doctor who suits you, but you may not have the time to search him out when you're suffering from the symptoms of hypoglycemia. Your first step has to be getting those symptoms checked out, even if it means going to a doctor you're not crazy about. See your current physician, a referral from a friend, or who-ever can fit you in at your local hospital. After an exam confirms that you're not suffering from something serious, such as a tumor, for example, you can then take your time to choose a healthcare provider who meets your needs and your expectations.

Knowing what to look for in a doc

Reactive hypoglycemia — the kind we discuss in this book — isn't life threatening by itself, although the symptoms and effects are known to seriously affect careers, relationships, and lives. Organic causes of hypoglycemia are a different story. Some of the underlying diseases or conditions can potentially be life threatening and can best be diagnosed during a thorough medical examination. (Check out Chapter 1 for more info.)

You have several things to consider when choosing a doctor:

✔ Familiarity with hypoglycemia (or at least being open-minded about it)

✔ Belief in the importance of nutrition for maintaining good health

✔ Willingness to work with alternative healthcare practitioners

✔ Taking your health complaints seriously

✔ Spending the time to thoroughly evaluate your condition

✔ Listening carefully to what you say

✔ Encouraging you to ask questions

✔ Asking you effective questions

✔ Explaining things clearly and fully

✔ Anticipating your health problems

✔ Welcoming your participation in the treatment

✔ Flexibility (no, not the kind that lets him do the splits)

Add anything else that's truly important to you to this list. The doctor's office location, the hospital where the doctor treats patients, and your health insurance may all factor into your consideration. Avoid anyone who's dismissive of you and your concerns. Drop him back into the swamp for further evolution. You deserve better than that.

More doctors are becoming open to discussion and treatment of conditions such as chronic hypoglycemia, which still isn't universally accepted as a valid diagnosis. Depending on your location, however, you may have to work to find these doctors. If you can't find a good doctor, you may consider going to a highly regarded alternative practitioner — but only after you've been cleared of organic causes of hypoglycemia. Always consult your physician before jumping to conclusions or consulting alternative healthcare practitioners.

Finding the right doc

After you know the qualities you want your doctor to have, develop a list of potential doctors in order to find the right doc for you. Keep the following steps in mind:

1. **Ask around.**

   Ask friends, coworkers, relatives, or any other health professionals you know who have been treated for hypoglycemia. If you don't know anyone who has hypoglycemia, contact a local medical society, church, or university medical center. (See the sidebar, "Cruise the Web for doctor-related matters" for online help.) Get several names, just in case the doctor you select isn't taking new patients or doesn't participate in your health insurance plan.

2. **When someone recommends a doctor, ask that person specific questions, such as:**

   • What is the doctor's area of expertise?

   • How would you describe the doctor's bedside manner?

   • What kind of experience did you have with the doctor?

3. **Set up an appointment just to chat with the doctor.**

   Make sure you both understand that you're trying to decide on a doctor. You'll have to pay for the visit, but you may save yourself some money in the long run. (See "Preparing Shows You're Caring [about Yourself]" later in this chapter for specific info.)

   During this call, ask the office about the doctor's fees, payment procedures, and insurance coverage.

Cruise the Web for doctor-related matters

When you're looking for the right doc to treat your hypoglycemia, you may be interested in seeing what you can find online. Some of the following Web sites actually direct you to doctors in your area, some provide contact and other info on alternative practitioners, and some give you hardcore scientific info:

✔ **American Association for Health Freedom** (www.apma.net): This association provides a political voice for healthcare providers who use a comprehensive approach, including nutritional therapies, preventive medical techniques, and natural treatments, when treating patients.

✔ **The American Association of Naturopathic Physicians (AANP)** (www.naturo pathic.org): This organization can help you find a naturopathic doctor. Naturopathic physicians treat hypoglycemia by finding the condition's underlying cause rather than by just focusing on your symptoms. The site offers resources and info about naturopathic medicine.

✔ **The American College for Advancement in Medicine** (www.acam.org): This society educates physicians in the advancements of preventive and nutritional medicine. The site features a book catalog, a database of doctors, a naturopathic physician directory, and membership info for doctors.

✔ **American Holistic Health Association (AHHA)** (www.ahha.org): This non-profit promotes the benefits of holistic principles. The site offers helpful resources, referral lists, self-help articles, and info about membership.

✔ **American Holistic Medical Association (AHMA)** (www.holisticmedicine. org): This association supports the professional and personal development of doctors as healers and educates them about the practice of holistic medicine. The site provides resources, links to other helpful Web sites, physician referrals, and membership info for doctors.

✔ **American Medical Association Doctor Finder** (http://webapps. ama-assn.org/doctorfinder/home.html): The AMA Web site offers doctor referrals, articles, and e-mail newsletters. The doctor finder page provides basic professional information on virtually every licensed physician in the United States. This page includes more than 690,000 doctors.

✔ **Holistic Online.com** (http://holisticonline.com): This site features conventional, alternative, integrative, and mind-body medicine.

✔ **National Health Information Center (NHIC)** (www.health.gov/nhic): This center was established in 1979 by the Office of Disease Prevention and Health Promotion (ODPHP), Office of Public Health and Science, Office of the Secretary, and U.S. Department of Health and Human Services. This site is a health information referral service. Health professionals and consumers who have health questions are put in touch with those organizations that are best able to provide answers for them.

✔ **Your Prescription for Health** (www.illnessisoptional.com): The site focuses on holistic health through its news blog, articles, "5 Steps to a Healthy Lifestyle" program, a holistic pharmacy, and a weekly radio show that's a forum for discussions about alternative medicine.

Dealing with doubters

Unfortunately, many doctors think that the only hypoglycemia that's legitimate is the type of low blood sugar that's induced by diabetics who miscalculate the amount of insulin they need. If you're suffering from a chronic condition of hypoglycemia that can't be traced to an obvious cause, your doctor may be tempted to dismiss your complaints. Should that happen, don't take it personally. Western medicine is used to treating illnesses aggressively with drugs and surgery rather than diet and lifestyle modifications.

Here are some reasons why a doctor may not believe hypoglycemia is causing your symptoms:

- ✔ Hypoglycemia has been rampantly overdiagnosed.

- ✔ Experts disagree on exactly what constitutes hypoglycemia.

- ✔ Glucose tolerance tests (GTT) for hypoglycemia (see Chapter 5) don't always show abnormally low levels of blood sugar.

- ✔ The array of symptoms are nonspecific (fatigue, dizziness, and depression, for example) and can have many different causes other than hypoglycemia.

- ✔ Patients can too easily ascribe everything to hypoglycemia, because it's associated with so many different symptoms.

- ✔ The symptoms associated with hypoglycemia can't be pinpointed to a specific dysfunction or damaged organs.

If your doctor doesn't believe you have hypoglycemia, but you're convinced that there's something physically wrong, then check out alternative practitioners who are more open to treating nonspecific health issues. (Check out "Putting Some Ohhhhmm into It: Alternative Medicine" later in this chapter.)

Choosing a Specialist

So, have you confessed everything to your kind doctor? Are you wondering whether you should see a specialist? Specialists offer many options. *Specialists* have at least three years of specialty training, under supervision, after getting their MD degree. Some specialists are primary care doctors, such as family physicians or *internists* (more on them in the next section). Other specialists concentrate on certain body systems, specific age groups, or complex scientific techniques.

A good way to find out about a doctor's expertise is to ask about her board certification. To be board certified after graduating from medical school, doctors have to pass an exam certifying them as specialists in certain fields of medicine. They also have to complete 150 hours of continuing medical education every three years and pass a comprehensive exam every seven years. (At least you know that they haven't forgotten everything they learned in med school.)

Is a specialist right for you? You're probably better off going to a doctor who already has your medical history first. Spend some time going over your symptoms and all your health concerns. Your doctor can direct you to the proper specialist should you need one. This section covers the main types of specialists that may help.

Internists and family doctors

Internists and family docs both can treat your hypoglycemia. So how do you know whether you need a specialist? The differences between an internist and a family physician are as follows:

- An *internist* is a doctor of adults who specializes in the diagnosis and treatment of nonsurgical ailments. You can find internists in hospitals and clinics. Some internists may specialize in other areas and become the friendly specialist that your illness calls for. These specialty areas may include arthritis, asthma, cancer, diabetes, and most surgical procedures.

- A *family doctor* is basically a general practitioner (GP) who has done residency in family practice. Family physicians provide healthcare to individuals regardless of their age. They give you regular check-ups, and they diagnose and treat most patient problems. You can visit a family doctor for a glucose tolerance test, which doctors sometimes use to screen for hypoglycemia. (See Chapter 5 to find out more about glucose tolerance tests.) Family physicians can refer you to another specialist if they can't treat certain problems.

If you're not sure what you have, or you suspect that you have hypoglycemia, internists or family docs are probably your best bet. Internists and family docs can schedule tests and refer you to hospitals and other specialists as needed. They discuss your treatment with your family (if appropriate) and anyone else involved in your healthcare. Their role is that of team leader.

Endocrinologists

Endocrinologists specialize in diseases and disorders of the endocrine system (hormones), which is involved in blood sugar regulation. Endocrinologists also treat diabetes, a condition that's connected to blood sugar regulation. In fact, both diabetics and hypoglycemics benefit from similar dietary restrictions and approaches (check out Chapter 6 for more info).

Should you see an endocrinologist if you think that you have hypoglycemia? Unless you have a glowing personal recommendation for an innovative endocrinologist with experience in hypoglycemia, an endocrinologist probably isn't your best bet. Why? Because, as specialists, endocrinologists are more familiar with serious illnesses and aren't usually attuned to identifying hypoglycemia's chronic conditions. If you want someone who's more attuned to hypoglycemia, go to your family doctor first.

You may consider seeing an endocrinologist, though, if you're obese, and you fail to lose weight after following the hypoglycemic food program for several months. (Keep a food journal to make sure that you're not subconsciously cheating! Flip to Chapter 6 to see how to keep a journal.) You may be suffering from other metabolic or hormonal imbalances. Endocrinologists are real pros at treating these conditions, as well as at identifying genetic or other factors (such as insulin resistance) that may be affecting your weight.

Preparing Shows You're Caring (About Yourself)

So you've talked to your friends, made a short list of potential doctors, and made an appointment with a prospective doctor. Before you head to the doctor's office, set aside 15–20 minutes a few days beforehand and plan ahead.

This section discusses what you need to take to your doctor's appointment and how to evaluate your doctor's visit to determine whether this doctor is right for you.

What to take to your appointment

Before you visit your doctor, make sure that you take the time to prepare for the visit. You can't just walk in and wing it. You're talking about your health right now, and you have the doctor's full attention, so make the most of it.

In order to have the most productive visit possible, prepare the following items before your first appointment:

✔ **A list of all your symptoms.** (Chapter 3 can help you in this arena.) Don't just leave your list of symptoms on the kitchen table; bring it with you! Chronic hypoglycemia can make you a wee bit forgetful, and the list can help jog your memory. You can show the doctor the list, but flesh out your symptoms by describing as completely as possible the timing, frequency, intensity, and duration of your problems.

When relating your symptoms, go from the general to the specific. Describe the following:

- How it feels, followed by facts that you can see or touch, such as body temperature

- When you first started to notice the symptom

- The time of the day that it occurs

- Whether you see a pattern

- How the various symptoms are affecting your life and work

✔ **Your medical history (including dates for surgeries, hospitalizations, and major illnesses) and your family's medical history.** Get copies of your medical records to show your doctor. (Most clinics have a medical history form for you to fill out. Bringing a copy of your medical records simplifies this procedure and ensures accuracy.)

Consult your family beforehand, so that you can construct as accurate and complete a medical history as possible. You may think that you know your family's medical history, but your parents or grandparents may have had illnesses that you aren't aware of. Grill your parents and siblings if you have to.

✔ **The names of medications you're taking and the dosage.** (Give either the generic or brand name, but skip any pet names you call them.) Your list should include any and all prescribed and *over-the-counter (OTC) meds* (medications you don't need a prescription for), vitamins, herbal supplements (see Chapter 7 for more on these treatments), and birth control. (Take samples of any herbs you're taking if you're unsure of the name. This is particularly true if you're also seeing a Chinese herbalist.)

✔ **Your food diary containing a record of everything you eat and any symptoms you have.** (Chapter 6 tells you how.) Showing what you've eaten may provide clues. However, don't expect your doctor to spend much time going over your diary. She'll likely just want a general idea. Some clinics provide you with forms that ask questions about your typical diet.

✔ **A list of any treatments that you're receiving from other practitioners.** These healthcare practitioners may include chiropractors, acupuncturists, dietitians, homeopaths, naturopaths, and osteopaths (but no psychopaths, please!).

✔ **A pen and paper for taking notes.** Jot down the most important points that your doctor covers, including advice or recommendations. Forgetting everything that was said is easy, especially when you're nervous. (When you find yourself nervous, take a few deep breaths to calm down.)

✔ **Insurance forms, cards, and other relevant data.** Many doctor's offices make copies of your insurance card and driver's license, and many billing departments won't file your claim unless you provide them with a form. Ask about what you need to bring before your appointment.

✔ **A list of any questions for your doc.** Ask your potential doctor these types of questions to see whether she's right for you:

- **Why do you think I'm having these problems?** Your doctor should be able to offer some explanations. If he brushes you off, or immediately decides what you have — without bothering to review your medical history or ask you relevant questions — find someone else.

- **If I don't have hypoglycemia, what do I have?** Be sure to take notes if your doctor suggests the names of other illnesses. If you don't know what they are, ask her.

- **When will you know what's causing the problem?** If the doctor directs you to take a battery of tests, then he'll wait for the results before he can accurately diagnose you.

- **Are you familiar with diagnosing and treating hypoglycemia patients?** If so, how many have you treated? Your doctor may not believe in hypoglycemia. If not, just make a mental note to yourself to find another health professional for this condition. All you're doing now is ensuring that you don't have problems other than hypoglycemia for which you should obtain medical treatment.

- **Do your patients with hypoglycemia improve with treatment?** Obviously, if the doctor doesn't believe that hypoglycemia is a clinical entity, then she's likely not even treating them.

- **What course of action do you plan on taking? What is the treatment plan?** No drugs can cure hypoglycemia. If the doctor recommends expensive treatment options, you should probably find another doctor.

- **What diet plan do you recommend?** If your doctor says that nutrition has no bearing or that you simply need to eat a balanced meal, you're seeing the wrong professional. Find someone with more expertise in hypoglycemia.

- **Can you refer me to a nutritionist, dietician, or other alternative healthcare practitioner (someone other than a doctor who practices traditional Western medicine)?** Chronic conditions such as hypoglycemia are better treated by alternative healthcare practitioners or doctors who practice integrative medicine. (These medical doctors are also proficient in alternative healthcare, such as acupuncture and herbal remedies.) Check out the "Putting Some Ohhhhmm into It: Alternative Medicine" section later in this chapter for more info.

In addition, coax a family member or friend into accompanying you to the visit. This person can prod your memory or provide more details about your illness, and she can give moral support to keep you on track if you get nervous. (Or kick you in the shin if you're not making any sense.) Oh, one more thing: No visit to the doctor is complete without nutritional snacks and reading materials (or quiet hand-held computer games).

Following up after the appointment

After the appointment, you want to figure out whether the doctor is a good fit. Ask yourself these questions:

- ✔ Did I feel comfortable with the doctor?
- ✔ Did I feel comfortable asking questions?
- ✔ Do I have confidence in this doctor?
- ✔ Did the doctor spend enough time answering all my questions?
- ✔ Did I actually understand what the doctor was saying? Did he explain things in terms I understand?

If you aren't reasonably satisfied, visit another doctor. If you feel okay about everything, schedule a complete physical exam. A complete exam includes tests for all your body's systems (cardiovascular, gastrointestinal, and more), as well as disease screenings. As you know, the doctor is going to take lots of things: a blood sample, urine and/or stool samples, and X-rays. Make sure to follow all instructions when preparing for the exam. If you're asked to refrain from eating or drinking anything other than water, do just as you're directed. If you don't follow your doctor's instructions, you can invalidate your test results.

Putting Some Ohhhhmm into It: Alternative Medicine

Two kinds of medical treatment can help alleviate your hypoglycemia. Earlier in this chapter, we talk about one kind: *allopathic (Western) medicine,* which targets specific illnesses with drugs and/or surgery. Allopathic treatment isn't always well-suited to addressing the numerous chronic complaints of a typical low blood-sugar sufferer. In almost all cases, the other kind of medical treatment — alternative or integrative medicine — may yield noticeable benefits beyond those available through conventional Western medicine.

This section focuses specifically on alternative medicine and how you can use it to treat your hypoglycemia. This section also discusses the many options available to you, including herbal medicine and acupuncture, and how you can use Western medicine and alternative medicine together to treat your hypoglycemia.

Defining your alternatives

Today, patients can benefit from many acceptable alternatives. The American Board of Holistic Medicine (ABHM) defines *holistic medicine* as "the art and science that addresses the whole person, body, mind and spirit." A holistic approach to treatment of hypoglycemia, with its focus on the interconnectedness of various factors (body, mind, emotional, social, and environmental) may be of great benefit as a supplement to conventional medical treatment, or even as a treatment in its own right.

In addition to viewing the mind and body as inseparable, alternative medicines use *noninvasive* (not requiring surgery), *nonpharmaceutical* (herbal or homeopathic remedies instead of prescription drugs) techniques. Many symptoms and conditions that are unresponsive to conventional treatment may yield to the application of nature's remedies. Although these techniques aren't yet accepted by most conventional medical doctors, an increasing number of such doctors are beginning to offer both allopathic and holistic approaches.

More insurance plans are beginning to cover alternative treatment approaches, but even if your insurance doesn't cover the alternative therapy you choose, selecting an alternative medicine practitioner can be worth the cost.

Considering your alternatives

So what alternatives can you consider? The alternatives are too numerous to list them all in this chapter. However, this section covers a few that we believe may be especially helpful for hypoglycemia.

Nutritional counseling

Much of the treatment for hypoglycemia revolves around food. As a result, you may want to consult a nutritional counselor or dietitian regarding possibilities for changing your diet or taking advantage of nutritional supplements.

A list of registered dietitians is available at the American Dietetic Association's Web site (www.eatright.org). Make sure the professional you consult is properly qualified and has a good track record for treatment of hypoglycemia. When choosing a dietitian or nutritionist, note that some professionals don't recognize chronic hypoglycemia as a bona fide diagnosis.

Herbal medicine

Herbal medicine is an alternative treatment that involves using supplements, powders, and actual raw herbs. Herbal medicine dates back to pre-history. People worldwide have used indigenous plants as remedies for illnesses. These are the three major approaches to herbal medicine:

- **Western:** The Western approach to herbal medicine has its roots in Greece and Rome. North American herbal medicine is based on European and Native American folk tradition. Plants or their extracts are used to treat specific symptoms and illnesses.

- **Indian (Ayurvedic):** Ayurvedic herbal medicine is part of Ayurvedic traditional medicine practiced in India for thousands of years. Patients are treated holistically as body, mind, and spirit. Herbs are used to balance the three main body types (Vata, Pitta, and Kappa). Because some Ayurvedic herbs may contain heavy metals at unsafe levels, go to a licensed Ayurvedic medical practitioner instead of buying OTC remedies.

- **Chinese:** Chinese herbal medicine is part of a centuries-old system of traditional Chinese medicine (TCM). Doctors prescribe herbs (preparations sometimes include minerals or animal products) to restore energy *(Qi)* balances. In China, herbs are used in state hospitals along with allopathic medicine.

Just because something is natural doesn't mean that it can't also be dangerous. Certain herbs don't go well when taken with prescription medicine. Consult your doctor before taking any herbal remedies. (For additional info on taking herbs, flip to Chapter 7.) And remember that herbs are meant to support you in your recovery — making the necessary dietary and lifestyle changes is still up to you. For hypoglycemics, the two pillars of recovery are diet (see Chapter 6 for specific recommendations on what to eat and what to avoid) and exercise (see Chapter 8 for tips on effective workouts).

Naturopathic medicine

Naturopathic medicine stresses health maintenance, disease prevention, and patient education and responsibility. It's not identified with any particular type of therapy; it's more a philosophy of life and health. You can find naturopathic doctors by visiting The American Association of Naturopathic Physicians Web site (www.naturopathic.org).

Orthomolecular psychiatry

Orthomolecular psychiatry is a treatment that's also called the *biochemical approach.* Orthomolecular psychiatry believes that when the brain is biochemically disorganized, so is the mind. It also believes in the existence of great individual differences in nutritional needs and metabolic processes. Doctors who practice this treatment use large, therapeutic doses of specific vitamins, nutrients, amino acids, trace elements, or fatty acids to achieve healing. They may also insist that you eliminate certain foods or food additives.

Acupuncture

An acupuncturist inserts very thin, sterile, stainless steel needles into points along the body's meridians. (*Meridians* are invisible channels that form the body's energy network.) Many acupuncturists also use *moxibustion,* a procedure in which *moxa* (a dry, yellow, fluffy material made from the herb mugwort) is rolled into a cone or a tiny ball, placed on a meridian acupoint, and lit.

Acupuncture not only helps ease hypoglycemic symptoms but it may also address the underlying blood sugar problem. To contact a qualified acupuncturist, ask for recommendations from a trusted physician or friend. You can also visit the American Academy of Medical Acupuncture Web site at www.medicalacupuncture.org.

Therapeutic massage and bodywork

Hands-on manipulation for healing is one of the oldest healing modalities in the world. Bodywork is an integral part of healthcare in many traditional cultures, most notably China and India. You can find some 80 different varieties of bodywork.

Depending on patient need and therapist orientation, a patient can take on a combination of massage and various types of structural integrative bodywork. Bodywork can

- ✔ **Reduce stress.** One of the proven effects of massage and bodywork is the release of *endorphins* — the happy hormones — and the reduction of stress hormones. Some studies suggest that stress may have as much of an impact on hypoglycemic symptoms as diet. But why is the release of stress and tension so good for people suffering from low blood sugar? Well, you end up with better blood circulation, which in turn improves the transportation of oxygen and nutrients throughout the body.

- ✔ **Ease physical pain.** Bodywork can also ease the sensation of physical pain — such as headaches and muscle stiffness — that can often accompany hypoglycemia.

Energy medicine

Energy medicine has hundreds of styles and schools. It's somewhat loosely defined as any healing approach whose underlying premise is that sickness and disease arise from imbalances in the vital energy field of the body. Practitioners work on clearing blocks to get the body's energies into a good flow, harmony, and balance. The aim is to promote overall health, vitality, and healing. Traditional Chinese medicine can be considered a form of energy medicine, because it views the body as an energy system (see the nearby sidebar "Releasing the qi with Chinese medicine"). One school of energy medicine that's rapidly gaining popularity is EFT (Emotional Freedom Technique). See Chapter 9 for the ways EFT can reduce stress.

The usefulness of energy medicine in the treatment of blood sugar imbalances is that it addresses the physical and emotional dysfunctions that are fairly typical manifestations of hypoglycemia. Another advantage is that patients can learn the many relatively simple energetic techniques for self-treatment. You can save time and money by treating yourself — and at your convenience — instead of relying only on other practitioners who may not always be available at the exact time that you need them. Energy medicine can be used in conjunction with medical practices, other alternative modalities, or as a complete system for self-care and self-help.

Working in tandem

Combining the Western and Eastern methods of healing may create the best of all worlds. This combination of methods may sound like something that's not easy to accomplish, but it's actually quite possible. For instance, the clinics run by Dr. Chow (the co-author

Releasing the qi with Chinese medicine

A growing body of research supports the benefits of traditional Chinese medicine (TCM). TCM particularly excels in conditions, such as chronic or nonspecific complaints, that Western medicine is weak at treating. All TCM practices are aimed at removing blockages to *qi* (or *chi,* or *energy*), as well as at restoring, rebalancing, and increasing the qi of an affected organ or organs.

What can you expect from a visit to a practitioner of TCM? He will carefully examine your face and tongue, take your pulse, perhaps feel your abdomen, and ask you detailed questions about your health, diet, lifestyle, and so on, before arriving at a diagnosis. The practitioner won't say that you're suffering from hypoglycemia. Instead, he may say, for instance, that you have too much dampness and cold in your body, and some stagnation in the kidney areas. In fact, two people with hypoglycemia can get different descriptions of what's ailing them, with the treatments varying accordingly. These differing diagnoses don't mean that the TCM doctors are wrong, or that what they're about to do doesn't have a prayer's chance of working. They simply mean that the causes of low blood sugar that are overlooked by Western doctors may be picked up by TCM practitioners, who view health through a different prism and attach different labels to dysfunctions of the body. TCM doctors can adjust herbal formulas in infinitesimal ways to fit your body's constitution. Similarly, with acupuncture, a practitioner can vary needling techniques and points of insertion to suit your body's requirements.

With TCM, some people see immediate improvement, while others don't. Realize that because TCM tries to get to the root of an illness, you may have to undergo many sessions before you see results. If you're interested in TCM, check your insurance plan to see whether it covers alternative healthcare, and make sure that the practitioner is licensed and certified.

of this book) offer *integrated treatments* to patients. Patients get regular physical check-ups and conventional Western medical care, which includes prescription medication, but they can also receive chiropractic, acupuncture, and Chinese herb treatments. The doctor can recommend alternative therapies that are appropriate for the patient, or the patient may ask for integrated treatment. These one-stop clinics are becoming more common in larger cities. Ask your healthcare practitioner for a referral.

If you don't have the opportunity to go to a one-stop clinic, however, make sure that your alternative medicine practitioners work with your primary physician. This way, you can avoid getting conflicting advice or having an important aspect of your health overlooked.

Here's some additional advice to consider when you're being treated with alternative medicine:

✔ **Don't try too many different therapies.** It'll be confusing and very expensive for you.

✔ **Avoid doctor-hopping.** Make sure that you give one doctor and one approach sufficient time to work for you.

✔ **Create a file for yourself.** Keep an accurate record of all your office visits, meds, vitamins, supplements, and anything else that you've been given, and take notes at each session. Your healthcare providers should be aware of everything you're doing in terms of your health.

Chapter 5

Getting the Lowdown on Low Blood Sugar

Perhaps you've been suffering from vague symptoms, like those we describe in Chapter 3, that you think may indicate hypoglycemia. Maybe you suspect that your body can't metabolize carbs properly. Or, maybe you're just the curious type. This chapter may provide a moment of truth: Here you find tools that help determine whether you have hypoglycemia. Following the guidelines in this chapter can help you make a good assessment of your symptoms. (Of course, see your doctor for the best assessment.)

Diagnosing hypoglycemia isn't as definitive as diagnosing diabetes. There's no absolute standard for determining hypoglycemia. You can take the glucose tolerance test (GTT), but it's not an infallible tool. Your doctor should also review your medical history and symptoms. In that sense, hypoglycemia is very much like other controversial diagnoses, such as chronic fatigue syndrome and fibromyalgia. (In fact, those syndromes may often be associated with low blood sugar; see Chapter 3 for more info.) Unfortunately, many people don't take hypoglycemia seriously. They see it as "the disease de jour" that hypochondriacs latch on to.

Taking the tests in this chapter doesn't substitute for seeing a doctor. Even if you test negatively here, see a doctor if you suspect that you have hypoglycemia or any other disorder.

Poking and Prodding Yourself

Before you gallivant to your doctor, you can prepare to see whether your symptoms truly indicate hypoglycemia. The best way to start is to take the questionnaire from this section. In addition, you may want to consider going on the trial diet later in the "Eating by trial" section, which can give you more info about your health, making it easier for your doctor to arrive at a diagnosis.

Filling in the circles: A questionnaire

Before you fill out the questionnaire, photocopy it, or leave yourself enough room to write down answers at a later date. Make sure that you write down the date you're taking the test; take the test every three weeks to keep track of your progress. All right, now you're primed and prepped. Answer Yes or No to the following:

Date:	Yes	No
Do you often crave sweets?		
Do you generally feel ravenously hungry between meals?		
Do you worry constantly or experience unprovoked anxieties?		
Do you have trouble sleeping?		
Are you irritable if you miss a meal?		
Do you feel tired, weak, or shaky if you miss a meal?		
Do you feel tired an hour or so after eating?		
Do you get dizzy when you stand suddenly?		
Do you experience vertigo (dizziness)?		
Do you usually feel fatigued or exhausted?		
Do you experience internal trembling?		
Are you often confused?		
Do you have heart palpitations?		
Do you get frequent headaches?		
Are you often forgetful?		
Do you have frequent crying spells?		
Do you have difficulty concentrating?		
Do you experience blurred vision?		
Do you have depression or mood swings?		

Date:	Yes	No
Do you feel as though you're going crazy?		
Do you have frequent backaches?		
Do you often have problems with digestion?		
Are you apt to engage in asocial or antisocial behavior?		
Are you indecisive?		
Do you get frequent leg cramps?		
Do you often experience muscle pains or muscular twitching?		
Do you often feel lightheaded?		
Do you experience numbness?		
Do you usually have cold hands and/or feet?		
Do you have fainting spells or blackouts?		
Do you have convulsions?		
Do you experience bloating?		
Are you overweight? (See the "Figuring out your BMI" sidebar to calculate.)		

Scoring: Add 1 for each Yes answer.

<5: Probably not hypoglycemic.

6 to 19: Hypoglycemia is likely.

>20: Hypoglycemia is extremely likely.

This test is a general guideline. If you have diabetics or hypo-glycemics in your family, you're probably prone to blood sugar imbalance and other manifestations of hypoglycemia. Even if you have only a few severe or recurrent symptoms, you may be hypo-glycemic. An excellent way to find out whether you're hypo-glycemic is to try this chapter's diet and see whether your symptoms diminish or clear. Following the diet gives your doc more info to work with.

See a doctor immediately if you have symptoms such as vertigo, blurred vision, numbness, blackouts, palpitations, or convulsions. These symptoms can indicate another, more urgent, health matter.

Figuring out your BMI

Calculating your *body mass index* (BMI), a number derived from your height and weight, is one generally accepted method of finding out whether you're overweight. People prone to blood sugar imbalances sometimes have a more difficult time keeping their weight under control. To calculate your BMI:

1. **Divide your body weight by 2.2.**

   For a 150-pound person: $150 \div 2.2 = 68.2$

2. **Divide your height in inches by 39.4.**

   For a person who is 5'8" (68 inches): $68 \div 39.4 = 1.7$

3. **Multiply your answer for step 2 by itself.**

   $1.7 \times 1.7 = 2.9$

4. **Divide the number from step 1 by the number from step 3.**

   Your final number is an estimation of your BMI. $68.2 \div 2.9 = 23.5$. This person's BMI is 23.5, which is in the healthy range.

In 1999, the National Institutes of Health issued these revised BMI guidelines:

✔ Below 18.5: Underweight

✔ 18.5 to 24.9: Healthy

✔ 25 to 29.9: Overweight

✔ 30 or greater: Obese

Bear in mind that BMI measurements for extremely muscular athletes and pregnant women aren't accurate.

Eating by trial

Trying out the following diet for at least 20 days can give you a fairly good indication of the likelihood of hypoglycemia. If you start feeling at least a bit better and some of your symptoms subside when you're on this diet, then chances are pretty good that you have low blood sugar. At this point, you may choose to get yourself tested (check out the next section), or simply embark on the hypoglycemia diet in Chapter 6.

✔ Avoid all sugars, stimulants, and heavy starch foods — this includes pasta, bread, corn, rice, and potatoes. (Be sure to read labels on everything, because prepared foods often contain hidden sugar.)

✔ Don't eat deep fried foods, breading, or sauces, and stay away from all desserts and fruits.

✔ Don't drink alcoholic beverages.

✔ If you smoke, try to at least cut back.

✔ You can eat as many vegetables as you like.

This diet is a test to help you find whether the seemingly unrelated symptoms you have are due to hypoglycemia, which is basically an underlying _metabolic disorder_ that makes your body incapable of handling carbs properly. (See Chapters 1 and 2 for more about what hypoglycemia is.) This diet isn't the prescribed diet for hypoglycemia (although similarities exist), and you don't have to stay on it forever. Your symptoms may temporarily worsen in the first week or so, but they should ease eventually.

Fill out the questionnaire in the previous section again at the end of the diet's trial period. If you have fewer symptoms, or if your symptoms become less intense or disappear, it's a good indication that you have hypoglycemia, particularly if you've already had all kinds of medical tests and nothing was found to be wrong.

As with any task worth doing, going on the trial diet may be challenging, but you can make it easier by exercising (see Chapter 8), using meditation and deep breathing techniques (see Chapter 9), and following Chapter 16's helpful hints for making life more manageable. In fact, you may be pleasantly surprised by how much better you feel and how much more energy you have.

Getting the 411 on Hypoglycemia Testing

We have some bad news: No lab tests can conclusively diagnose hypoglycemia. That's because of the controversy over the criteria for evaluating the test. Looking only at blood sugar values can give skewed results, flagging healthy people as hypoglycemics; and conversely, hypoglycemics may be told they're healthy — the latter is a scenario that happens all too frequently. People commonly spend hundreds or even thousands of dollars on tests that tell them nothing conclusive. Some doctors may question whether your so-called symptoms are just in your head. And some people have hypo symptoms even with their lowest numbers in the normal range.

Despite the drawbacks, doctors can use lab tests as part of the diagnostic procedure. Two tests can help diagnose hypoglycemia: the glucose tolerance test (GTT) and glucose insulin tolerance test (G-ITT).

Although the GTT can diagnose diabetes and hypoglycemia, these days, many doctors don't even consider it the instrument of choice for diagnosing hypoglycemia. The G-ITT is a standard GTT coupled with the measurement of insulin levels; it's much more sensitive in spotting faulty sugar metabolism. Studies show that people with suspected diabetes or hypoglycemia who test normal when only the GTT is taken show up as abnormal on the G-ITT.

This section takes a closer look at these tests and the pros and cons of your doctor conducting these tests. Furthermore, this section walks you through the actual tests so you know what to expect, and then it helps you interpret the results.

The pros and cons of these tests

The advantages to taking either the GTT or the G-ITT, should the results indicate that you have an abnormality, include the following:

- ✔ If you need to convince your employer or your family and friends that your hypoglycemia isn't all in your head, you have medical documentation for proving your case. (See Chapter 11 for more about work.)

- ✔ The test is likely to motivate you to make dietary changes.

- ✔ You can use the results to predict when your blood sugar will dip, and then you can schedule your snacks accordingly. (For instance, you can try eating 20 minutes before the predicted blood sugar drop.)

- ✔ The test can indicate whether you need further testing to determine whether you have a serious organic cause for your hypoglycemia, such as a tumor of the pancreas. Chances are that you don't have cancer of the pancreas, because it's a rare condition, but ruling out other causes is always a good idea.

The GTT (and G-ITT) is no picnic in the park. It's long, it's stressful, and for those of you who have a severe case of hypoglycemia, your symptoms will probably flare up during the test. When given the GTT or G-ITT, some people may have hypoglycemic symptoms even though their blood sugar level falls comfortably within the normal range. An individual may go totally nuts and yet have a virtually identical glucose tolerance test reading to someone who's calm and collected. Results that are considered normal may not necessarily be normal for you. Your body may not be able to function properly with a blood sugar level that doctors consider normal.

If you want to spare yourself the time and expense of taking the tests, just try out the two-week trial diet in this chapter. Many hypoglycemia veterans attest that how you feel while you're on the diet gives you at least as good a clue to whether you're hypo-glycemic as the tests do.

What to expect from the tests

Before you take either the GTT or the G-ITT, find out whether your insurance will pick up the cost. Most insurance policies cover GTTs for diabetics; they may also reimburse you if your doctor confirms a diagnosis of hypoglycemia. But unless you're enrolled under a generous policy, chances are that you'll have to pay out-of-pocket.

If you and your doctor decide that one of the glucose tolerance tests is right for you, the following sections walk you through the tests so you know what to expect.

Surfing to find more testing info

When you're wondering whether you have hypoglycemia, or if you've been recently diagnosed, you may be curious about the tests your doctor will do, or has done. The following Web sites explain a bit more about different types of testing your doctor may perform:

✔ **Genova Diagnostics** (`www.gdx.net`): This lab, which was formerly named the Great Smokies Diagnostic Laboratories, can perform food-allergy tests. The Web site offers information about the different tests the laboratory performs, news about the latest lab developments, educational resources, an online book-store, and a newsletter.

✔ **Health Equations** (`www.healthequations.com`): This site provides nutri-tional blood testing and information about the testing, as well as articles on topics such as cholesterol and heart disease.

✔ **Reactive Hypoglycemia Home Page** (`www.fred.net/slowup/hypo.html`): This home page gives you information about treatments that can help relieve the symptoms of hypoglycemia. It also provides a good list of resources for those who want to find out more about the condition.

Pretest

The glucose tolerance tests are usually conducted in the morning, after you've *fasted* (gone without food) for 10 to 12 hours. Ask a friend or family member to take you to the clinic and pick you up after the test. Because you may have severe reactions to the test, driving home or taking public transportation can be dangerous.

Keep the following in mind:

✔ Tell your doctor about any prescription meds you're currently taking, especially diuretic drugs, anti-epileptic drugs, contraceptives, and drugs containing cortisone or aspirin.

✔ Arrange to have extra blood samples taken while you're having obvious symptoms, such as rapid pulse, sweating, or sudden weakness, at least 15 minutes before the next blood sample is drawn. When you get these symptoms, call a nurse immediately.

✔ Arrange to get a personal copy of your results.

✔ Make sure that you get the six-hour test and not the shorter three-, four-, or even five-hour test. For some individuals, blood sugar may not fall below the normal level until after the fourth or fifth hour. Yes, this means that the test will be an all-day affair. Here's what you should prepare:

- Good reading materials (for helping pass the time)

- Food to eat when the test is over (to help level out your blood sugar)

- A notebook or some papers (to help pass the time; also good for adding to your food journal later)

- A pen (because trying to write with crayons is tough)

- A watch (so you can record your body's rhythms and see the light at the end of the testing tunnel)

More blood? Sure, we'll take it

You can ask for blood to be drawn every half hour to increase the accuracy of the test, but the test will cost more — and you'll have many more lovely puncture wounds on your arms. Something to consider: Instead of having your blood tested every half hour, make a special request to have a specimen taken after 3½ hours. (It's not normally done, so you have to ask.) This specimen can reveal abnormalities that may be missed otherwise.

You can't touch any food until the test is over. If you do, the results are invalidated. You can drink only water.

During the test

So you have on your comfy clothes, you're clutching a new book, and your tummy is rumbling. Here's what to expect when you show up at the clinic:

1. **Blood is drawn to take a *baseline blood sugar measurement* (the amount of sugar in your bloodstream after an overnight fast).**

   The doctor needs to have a baseline measurement in order to find out what your body does with the sugar. If the thought of needles freaks you out, refer to Chapter 9 and practice some of the stress-relieving exercises.

2. **You're given a glucose solution to drink.**

   It's presented in a bottle containing about 75 grams of glucose (sugar) in 300 ml (milliliters) of water. You don't have to drink it in one gulp, but you want to swallow it reasonably quickly; don't nurse it like a cup of latte. You drink only this one bottle.

   Don't lie down during the test unless you're very weak. Blood sugar tends to remain high if you don't move at all, so lying down may skew the results. If possible, walk around the clinic and stretch out your legs. Just get back in time for the blood draw.

3. **Blood is drawn again at 30 minutes and at 1 hour, and then hourly for up to 6 hours.**

   The blood samples are examined for their actual sugar content at specific intervals. The samples show how your body utilizes sugar.

4. **You're informed when the test is over.**

5. **You're told the results after your doctor gets them from the lab.**

Some patients experience vertigo, disorientation, and other severe symptoms during the test, although none of these are common. Some start crying uncontrollably, get into an argument with the nurse, or otherwise engage in bizarre behavior. If you experience any of these symptoms, don't be alarmed.

Write down any symptoms or adverse effects that you experience during the test, such as dizziness, abdominal cramps, irritability, depression, and so on, and the time that they occurred. Keeping track of this info is crucial, because it can aid in interpreting your test results. You'll be able to compare the reactions that you experienced during the test to your blood sugar levels at the time of the reactions. This is a good reason to have someone there with you: Your companion can note such incidences, even if you're too far gone to write anything down.

Post-test

You're done. Take a breath. You'll probably be tired after the test, so don't schedule anything demanding that night. You may want to skip your kickboxing class. Of course, if you're feeling bright and chipper and raring to go, don't hold back. Go challenge the neighborhood wrestling champ if you want. As long as it's legal, feel free to do whatever you like.

How your doc interprets the results

To interpret the results of the GTT or the G-ITT test, you need to understand how doctors measure the amount of sugar in the blood. Results are shown per 100 milliliters (ml) of blood. Here are the spans for fasting blood sugar levels:

- ✔ **80–110 mg:** The normal span
- ✔ **110–125 mg:** Impaired glucose tolerance
- ✔ **>126 mg:** Raises the suspicion of diabetes

After you swallow the glucose drink, you're no longer considered to be fasting. The blood sugar level rises slightly in the healthy individual, perhaps to 120 mg, depending on where the fasting level was, and then falls back to the fasting level. For a short period of time, the blood sugar level drops slightly below the level it was at during fasting, and then it returns to normal fairly quickly.

The nonfasting blood sugar levels are recorded after 30 minutes and then every hour after you drink the glucose beverage:

- ✔ **<140 mg:** Normal
- ✔ **140–199 mg:** Impaired glucose tolerance
- ✔ **>200 mg:** Indicates diabetes

In the diabetic person, blood sugar comes down very slowly, returning to the fasting level after six or more hours. And what about hypoglycemics? Unfortunately, the criteria for diagnosing hypoglycemia aren't so clear. Doctors can't agree on a specific number. However, hypoglycemia is officially recognized in an individual only if fasting blood sugar falls below 45 mg during a 72-hour fast. Some doctors adopt more stringent diagnostic criteria called the *Whipple triad*. The patient must satisfy the following requirements before she can be formally diagnosed as hypoglycemic:

✔ The glucose levels must fall to less than 40 mg.

✔ Symptoms of hypoglycemia.

✔ The hypoglycemic symptoms must be reversed when the glucose levels are returned to normal.

To make an accurate assessment of either the GTT or the G-ITT, your doctor should observe how fast your blood sugar drops (rather than how low it drops). Basically, hypoglycemia is suspected if the natural rise is followed by a rapid drop below the normal fasting range. The lower and faster it drops, the more severe the condition. A person may experience more problems if his sugar level drops from 200 mg to 100 mg in one hour or less, than if it drops from 100 mg to 45 mg in two or three hours.

So, when diagnosing hypoglycemia, consider these factors:

✔ How fast does the blood sugar level return to normal?

✔ How long does the sugar level remain at the low point?

For instance, the blood sugar level may drop to a low 45, but if it recovers quickly and returns to the fasting level in about an hour, you may not even notice it, or you may experience only mild symptoms. You may have more severe symptoms if, say, your blood sugar drops to 65 mg and remains there for a few hours because it takes a long time to return to your fasting level.

G-ITT this test

In addition to testing your glucose level, we strongly recommend that you have your insulin or epinephrine level measured at the same time (via the G-ITT), because hypoglycemic symptoms often correlate better with elevations of these hormones than with blood sugar levels. People with hypoglycemia often have food sensitivities that can contribute to their symptoms, but lab tests for food sensitivities can be quite expensive. And because there's so much disagreement about how valid they are, use the elimination diet. It may clue you in on which foods are causing your problems.

Even if you don't meet the official criteria to be diagnosed as hypo-glycemic, you may still experience all the adverse effects due to your body's inability to metabolize carbohydrates properly.

Because hypoglycemics have so many different sugar curves, you should select a doctor who is specifically trained to treat hypo-glycemia. (Chapter 4 has info on selecting the right doctor.)

Figure 5-1 shows what a hypoglycemic's curves may look like.

- ✔ Line A shows that the glucose level has fallen below 50 mg.
- ✔ Line B indicates that the level has fallen below the original fasting level of 80 mg.
- ✔ Line C shows a severe percentage drop in the short term.
- ✔ Line D stays above the fasting level of 100 mg for an extended time.

Graphing your own results

By graphing your own results, you get a pictorial representation of exactly when your blood sugar falls. Your doctor doesn't usually give you a graph; she just tells you the results. If you have a graph, it's easier to see just when your blood sugar falls. Also, if you need to convince someone that you have hypoglycemia, something visual works better than using just words to explain.

After you have a GTT test performed

1. **Ask your doctor to give you a copy of the results of your test.**

2. **Chart a graph.**

   You can see examples in Figures 5-1, 5-2, 5-3, 5-4, and 5-5.

3. **Compare the notes you took during the test to your blood sugar levels represented on the graph.**

4. **Go over the results with your doctor.**

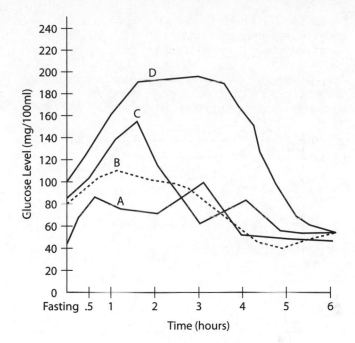

The following are considered hypoglycemic curves:

A: Glucose level falls below 50mg/dl.

B: Glucose level falls more than 30mg below fasting level.

C: Glucose level shows severe percentage drop in short time.

D: Glucose level stays above fasting level for extended period.

Figure 5-1: Curves for hypoglycemia.

One picture is worth 1,000 words, so one graph should be good for at least 500. Figures 5-2 through 5-5 offer four sample graphs that give you an idea of what the tests look like. See just how sexy these glucose tolerance curves can be? You can tell how the rise and fall of the blood sugar level for diabetes, relative hypoglycemia, and flat glucose tolerance (considered a type of hypoglycemia) differ significantly from one another.

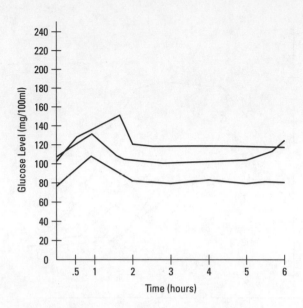

Figure 5-2: Normal glucose tolerance curves.

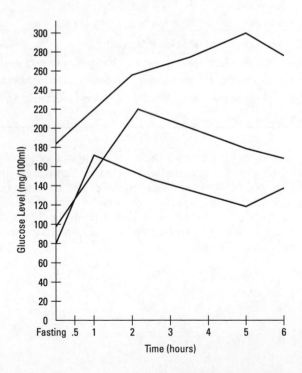

Figure 5-3: Glucose tolerance curves for diabetes.

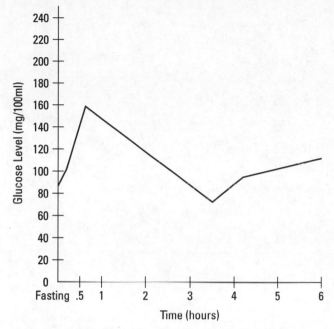

Figure 5-4: Relative hypoglycemia: The glucose level falls 50mg or more below fasting levels in one hour.

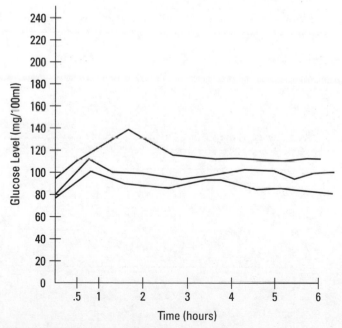

Figure 5-5: Flat glucose tolerance curves.

Chapter 6

Gorging on Good Health

· ·

In This Chapter

▶ Understanding the importance of nutrition

▶ Following a specific diet plan

▶ Determining proper serving sizes

▶ Sticking with your vegetarian diet

▶ Keeping a food journal

· ·

*Y*ou may not know it yet, but the road to radiant health is paved with good foods. Granted, these foods may not be your number one preference right now, but as you make your way through this book, your palate and your taste buds will likely change.

Thankfully, treating hypoglycemia is directly linked to changing your diet. Vitamins and dietary supplements can help (see Chapter 7 for a complete list), but you don't need expensive medication to get results. Making changes to your diet does, however, take work and commitment. Only you can make the day-to-day changes required to turn your health around. But as you do so, you'll be heartened by the vitality you experience as you recover from the lifestyle that made you ill. (For more on the concept of recovery, see Chapter 1.)

Depending on where you live, you may not find some of the foods mentioned in this chapter in regular grocery stores. You can, however, easily obtain them in natural food stores or large, international grocery stores. If you can't find them, check out the "Using the Web to help you eat healthy" sidebar in this chapter.

As you embark on your eating plan, try to think in terms of abundance rather than restriction and limitation. Creating a food plan that takes your biochemical individuality into account helps you achieve optimum health. This chapter looks at the importance of eating well and can help you develop an eating plan.

Of Food Pyramids and Healthy Eating

Do you often get strong cravings for something sweet or starchy: a candy bar, a bagel, mashed potatoes? Your low blood sugar is driving you toward something that will give you a boost of energy. If you cave into your cravings, you can set off a chain of reactions that culminates in a *blood sugar crash* — when the blood sugar level falls below the optimum range in which the body functions.

The fact is that food with white sugar and white flour is absolutely the worst for blood sugar control. (Check out Chapter 2 for the scoop on how your body reacts when you eat carbs.) This section explains the food pyramid and guides you to healthier eating.

Re-designing the familiar pyramid

Many Americans try to eat healthy by eating a high-carb, low-fat, and low-protein diet or a high-protein, low-carb diet — or whatever diet happens to be the most popular. Part of the blame falls on the old food pyramid recommended by the U.S. Department of Agriculture (USDA) and on diet gurus who make extravagant weight loss claims.

Most Americans are familiar with the old food pyramid. At the base of the old pyramid were grains, such as rice, wheat, oats, and cereals. The USDA recommended six to eleven servings a day of this group. Moving upward, the next section featured fruits (two to four servings) and vegetables (three to five servings). The third section had dairy products, meats, poultry, fish, eggs, dry beans, and nuts (two to three servings). At the very top were the fats, oils, and sweets, which were to be consumed sparingly.

The new dietary guidelines for Americans that were introduced in 2005 better reflect current nutritional findings, but still remain inadequate, especially for hypoglycemics. The revised pyramid allows you to eat up to half of your total grain intake in the form of refined starch, and lets you eat sweets. Moreover, it lumps fruit juices together with fruits. But fruit juices lack the fiber and minerals in whole fruits that slow down the release of blood sugar and help the body absorb the sugar contained in fruits. Fruit juices are therefore *not* the same as whole fruits, and are off limits to anyone suffering from hypoglycemia.

As you can see, the USDA diet — the old one or the new one — is a no-no for the hypoglycemic person, because the consumption of sweets and refined starch can set off a yo-yo blood sugar syndrome. (You can partially offset this yo-yo effect by eating enough fat and protein, but that may add up to way too many calories! Anyway, too many carbs aren't good for you.) Many people who go too low on fats and protein experience the following problems:

- Constant hunger
- Cravings for starch and sugar
- Deficiencies in calcium and vitamins A, D, E, and K
- A liver impairment for dealing with toxins

Despite these flaws, the USDA's revised food pyramid is an improvement over the old one because it shows a swath of six-colored rays that indicate food groups to emphasize and to minimize, instead of a fixed number of servings in each food group, which doesn't take into account individual differences. The pyramid also stresses the importance of exercise by drawing a person running up the steps of the pyramid.

To help stabilize your blood sugar, eat some protein with every meal or snack. (An exception to this rule is fruits. Some people experience digestive discomfort when they mix fruit with protein. Not everyone does, so experiment and see what works best for you.) Carbs affect your blood sugar the most, because they're easily digested and transformed into glucose. By contrast, protein is digested much slower. Eating some protein slows digestion and helps stabilize blood sugar. When it comes to your blood sugar, carbs really count. (We provide a list of foods that contain protein later in this chapter.)

Building a hypoglycemic pyramid

If you're hypoglycemic, and you want a healthy diet, just reshape the old pyramid a bit as shown in Figure 6-1. Hypoglycemics have their very own food pyramid! We use the old one as a model rather than the new one, because the colored rays representing the different food groups aren't as easy to take in at a glance. MyPyramid depends on the Web site for details and an interactive computer game to help users understand the food recommendations. We'd rather keep things as simple as possible.

So, at the base are fresh fruits and vegetables (more veggies than fruits). The next section contains high-quality, low-fat protein (lean cuts of beef or skinless chicken). These two groups should fill up most of the pyramid. Dairy is there, if you can tolerate dairy. Stick to two to three servings. Near the top are breads, grains, and pasta, which are to be seldom eaten. Fats and oils occupy the uppermost, narrow portion of the pyramid. The majority of your carb needs are met by fresh, nutrient-dense fruits and leafy-green veggies.

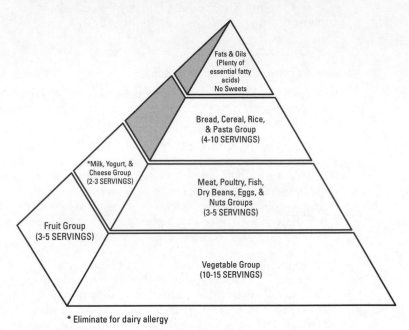

Fats & Oils
(Plenty of essential fatty acids)
No Sweets

Bread, Cereal, Rice, & Pasta Group
(4-10 SERVINGS)

*Milk, Yogurt, & Cheese Group
(2-3 SERVINGS)

Meat, Poultry, Fish, Dry Beans, Eggs, & Nuts Groups
(3-5 SERVINGS)

Fruit Group
(3-5 SERVINGS)

Vegetable Group
(10-15 SERVINGS)

* Eliminate for dairy allergy

Figure 6-1: This pyramid is for the hypoglycemic.

If you use this hypoglycemic food pyramid as your guide, keep the following things in mind:

✔ Carbohydrates should comprise 40 to 60 percent of your total calories. Nutritionally speaking, eating complex carbs (whole wheat bread) is better than eating simple carbs (white bread). But before you go on an eating spree of all-organic, all-natural, whole-wheat cakes and breads, consider this: Even complex carbs have the tendency to raise your blood sugar and trigger excess insulin production. Restrict your total carbohydrate intake. And if you're at all wheat sensitive, you have to elimi- nate wheat-based foods, such as bread and pasta. (Flip to Chapter 3 for details on food sensitivities.)

✔ Protein should comprise 15 to 30 percent of your total calo- ries. Remember, though, that although protein occupies a sig- nificant portion of your diet, it should by no means outstrip your carbohydrate intake. Aim for regular and consistent pro- tein intake, not a high protein intake.

✔ Unless your doctor puts you on a special diet, you should strive to get about 15 to 20 percent of your calories from fats.

Keeping your diet in balance

The key to using the modified food pyramid for hypoglycemia is keeping things balanced. Here are some clues that you may be getting too much or too little of the different food groups and what you can do to fix the situation.

Too much protein, too few carbs

Depending on body size, the maximum amount of protein a person can tolerate is about 200 to 300 grams a day. If you experience the following symptoms, you're most likely eating too much protein and not enough carbs:

- Nervousness
- Irritability
- Jitters
- Overall feeling of weakness
- Compulsion to overeat

If you do experience these symptoms, they'll most likely clear up in a few days (several weeks at most) after you add carbs to your diet.

Too much protein can pose these health problems:

- Damage to the liver, kidneys, and brain
- Calcium deficiency
- Gouty arthritis (a painful condition of the joints caused by excess uric acid in certain tissues)

Too little fat (believe it or not)

Most people love fat. And no wonder — fat gives foods a pleasant mouth feel and can taste pretty good too. Just look at the industry sales of high-fat ice creams and other fatty foods like chips and French fries. Although too much fat is unhealthy and can lead to weight gain if consumed in excess, in general, fats

- Help your body function properly
- Slow down the rate at which carbs enter your bloodstream
- Give you the feeling of being full
- Release a hormone that signals your brain to stop eating

If you're hypoglycemic and you don't consume enough fat (about 15 to 20 percent of your diet), you may start craving starches and run the risk of eating too much. But wait! Don't run out just yet for your favorite fast food fix. First read the "The squeaky hypoglycemic gets the grease: Fats" section for more info.

Shunning problematic foods

Food has the ability not only to make you sick but also to heal. In the case of hypoglycemia, the key to successful treatment is through the elimination — not the addition — of certain foods. Avoiding foods that wreak havoc on your system has the greatest impact on your health — as much impact as (or more than) what you eat or what supplements you take.

This section includes a list of foods and beverages that you should avoid. After you follow this outline for awhile and your body becomes stronger, you can expand your diet and even cheat occasionally. When you're transitioning to a healthier diet, be as careful as possible. If you usually inhale the typical Western diet, many familiar foods (perhaps your all-time favorites) may be included in the huh-uh list. Don't despair, though. You don't have to follow the recovery program perfectly for it to work.

These are the foods that you should shun:

- ✔ Sugar (including white, brown, raw, and turbinado).

- ✔ Refined flour (white, bleached, unbleached, and enriched) and everything made from it. Generally speaking, if it looks white, it's white flour! Read labels, avoiding anything not made from whole grains. And don't be misled by white bread colored brown masquerading as whole wheat. Wheat flour, for instance, contains refined flour. If the first ingredient doesn't say whole wheat, the bread goes back on the shelf.

- ✔ Polished rice (white rice) and any kind of instant rice.

- ✔ Processed proteins (lunchmeats, sausages, bacon, hot dogs — anything with additives or preservatives).

- ✔ Processed cheese (cheese made by combining one or more natural cheeses with an emulsifying agent, and then heating and mixing it; American cheese is processed).

- ✔ Coffee, black tea, and anything else with caffeine (including chocolate).

- ✔ Soft drinks (carbonated drinks, including all colas).

- ✔ Alcohol.

✔ MSG (monosodium glutamate). Everyone, but especially meta-
bolically sensitive individuals like hypoglycemics, should
avoid this seasoning. Other names for MSG include hydrolyzed
protein, caseinate, soy extract, yeast extract, meat tenderizer,
Accent, and Ajinomoto.

The World's Your Oyster and Your Pear — Foods to Eat

After checking the list of foods to avoid, you may feel that you're
forced to make the grim choice of either never enjoying eating
again, or living the rest of your life in compromised health. In fact,
you don't have to do either. Eating a wide variety of foods — within
the constraints of your hypoglycemic diet — ensures that you're
getting the proper balance of vitamins and minerals (which we discuss in depth in Chapter 7).

Most people forget that healthy food is also truly good-tasting
food. You can eat lots of delicious foods; moreover, when you
embark on your recovery program, unhealthy foods start losing
their appeal. Although you may always hear the siren call of your
favorite forbidden foods, it becomes more muted over time;
besides, you'll have so much more zest for life that you'll want to
get right back on course. This section looks at the healthful foods
that you want to eat to lessen your hypoglycemia symptoms.

Darned if you do, darned if you donut

Donuts and danishes spell disaster when it comes to your blood sugar. Muffins (even
if they're low-fat) and bagels, which seem to be healthy alternatives, spike your
blood sugar just as high and just as rapidly. This is also true for most breakfast cereals (if you're going to eat sugar-coated cereal, you may as well have a candy bar)
and *muesli,* a Swiss breakfast cereal consisting of rolled oats, nuts, and fruits.

Health food stores carry all sorts of cereals that actually contain some good vitamins,
but these, too, are best avoided, especially in the early days of your recovery. If you
do eat these types of cereal, make sure that you choose the ones that have no added
sugar of any sort, no additives, and lots of fiber. Slow-cooked oatmeal is a healthy
choice, particularly if you throw in some crunchy, protein-rich nuts or seeds. (Steer
clear of instant oats and other instant foods, which convert almost instantly into blood
glucose.) *Steel cut oats* — the inner portion of the oat kernel — are best. They contain more nutrients, because they're less processed than quick, instant, or rolled oats.
Steel cut oats, which are also called Scotch oats or Irish oatmeal, are chewier, have
more texture, and are slower to cook. They're available at health food stores.

Life's a bowl of cherries: Fruits

Fruits are yummy, not to mention rich in nutrients and all kinds of beneficial compounds. And they're just the thing to eat if you want something sweet.

The sugar in fruit is called *fructose,* and it appears that fructose doesn't cause as rapid a rise in blood sugar as simple sugars. Fructose has to be changed to glucose in the liver before it can be used by the body, so the rise in your blood sugar is more moderate when you eat fruits. The fiber in fruits also helps keep the blood sugar from rising too quickly. Besides, fruits can help control sugar cravings (instead of triggering them, like processed snacks do). In addition, fruits have vitamins, minerals, and enzymes that aid in digestion. But don't consume fructose alone, without the fruit, because then it's almost as bad as table sugar.

Using the Web to help you eat healthy

Are you chomping at the bit, looking for more info about eating healthy and beating your hypoglycemia? Obviously we have only so many pages in this book to provide you with helpful info. If you want more in-depth facts, we suggest you check out the following Web sites:

✔ **American Dietetic Association (www.eatright.org):** This Web site provides a nationwide dietitian referral service, information and tips for maintaining good nutrition, listings of good resources, a catalog of products and services, and membership information for doctors and students.

✔ **Celiac Disease and Gluten-free Diet Support Center (www.celiac.com):** This center provides resources and information for people with special dietary needs, particularly those suffering from celiac disease, gluten intolerance, dermatitis herpetiformis, or wheat allergy. It also offers gluten-free and wheat-free online resources.

✔ **Home of the glycemic index (www.glycemicindex.com):** The official Web site of the Glycemic Index and GI Database provides a search function to find the glycemic index and glycemic load of any given food, and supplies a newsletter, GI testing, database, books, news releases, and general information related to the GI.

✔ **nSpired Natural Foods (www.nspiredfoods.com):** This Web site offers a variety of natural (and/or organic) foods, including Pumpkorn, an all-natural snack food made from pumpkin seeds.

✔ **Nutrition Database (www.nutritiondata.com):** This site analyzes the nutritional content of foods. You can find the calories, protein, carbohydrate, fat, and fiber content of most foods by using the site's search engine.

✔ **Shake Off the Sugar** (www.shakeoffthesugar.net): This Web site provides info, recipes, and products for cooking without sugar. It also features tools for determining the nutritional, protein, and sugar content of common foods.

✔ **Sugar Shock** (www.sugarshock.com): Connie Bennett, journalist and author of *Sugar Shock!,* provides support in helping people kick the sugar habit. The site offers an e-zine, testimonials, and sundry products.

✔ **USDA Food and Nutrition Information Center** (fnic.nal.usda.gov): This Web site provides info about food, nutrition, and food safety. It also offers a large variety of resources, links, and databases that deal with nutrition.

✔ **Vegetarian Lowcarb (Immune Web)** (immuneweb.org/lowcarb): The Vegetarian Lowcarb section of this site shows vegetarians how to follow a low-carb diet. It provides info on low-carb vegetable protein sources, products, menus, recipes, a mailing list, and links to other good resources.

✔ **Vegetarian Resource Group (VRG)** (www.vrg.org): This nonprofit organization focuses on educating the public about vegetarianism and related issues, such as health, nutrition, ecology, ethics, and world hunger. The Web site offers recipes, a newsletter, links to other good Web sites, a bulletin board, excerpts from the *Vegetarian Journal,* and an online catalog.

✔ **The Yeast Connection** (www.yeastconnection.com): This organization provides support for patients suffering from candida overgrowth. You can get expert advice by e-mailing questions to Dr. Carolyn Dean, medical advisor to the Yeast Connection, and author of more than a dozen books, including *IBS For Dummies* (Wiley). She's also available for fee-for-service telephone health consultations. Free weekly e-news and a yeast-fighting program are also available from the site.

The preferred fruits for hypoglycemics are of the not-too-sweet variety:

✔ Apples

✔ Cherries

✔ Grapes

✔ Guava

✔ Kiwi

✔ Papaya

✔ Pears

✔ Strawberries

Fruits to avoid, especially when you're in the initial stages of recovery, include the following:

✔ Bananas

✔ Dates

✔ Figs

✔ Raisins and other dried fruits (After you're feeling better, you may occasionally eat small amounts after soaking them in water or cooking with cereal. As a general rule, avoid dried fruits.)

If you have digestive problems associated with eating fruits with your meals, try eating fruit half an hour before a meal, or two to three hours afterward. Fruit contains a lot of fiber, so it shouldn't cause a blood sugar spike even if you eat it by itself. (Melons don't seem to combine well with other foods or even other fruits. Eat melons by themselves, separately from other foods.)

Try fruits that have a lower glycemic index (GI), because they won't raise your blood glucose as much. (Check out `www.glycemicindex.com` for a list of fruits with a low GI.) If even the low GI fruits seem to give you trouble, skip fruits altogether; some hypoglycemics in the earliest part of recovery can't metabolize them properly.

Vegging out isn't a bad thing

Your mother was right: You need to eat your veggies. Do you want to be free of distressing hypoglycemic symptoms? Eat your vegetables. Do you want to combat aging and look and feel young for as long as possible? Eat your vegetables. Do you want your brain to remain sharp, clear, and focused? Eat your vegetables.

Vegetables carry a greater nutritional wallop than most man-made vitamins or supplements. They're chock full of vitamins, minerals, protein, high-quality carbs, essential fatty acids, antioxidants, fiber, and a host of other health-promoting substances that scientists are only beginning to unravel. Veggies, especially green ones, are a real boon for people battling blood sugar imbalance because they're rich in essential fatty acids, such as Omega-3 oils. Vegetables are blood sugar neutral, meaning they don't trigger increases in insulin or blood sugar.

Eating the best veggies in the best state (raw, that is)

Always try to eat fresh vegetables in their raw state, because cooking destroys some of the nutrients. On the other hand, some

vegetables, such as asparagus, cauliflower, and cabbage, may promote better digestion when *lightly* cooked. Raw spinach can interfere with calcium absorption, so if you do eat it raw, make sure that
you don't consume it with calcium-rich foods. For variety, you can
steam, sauté, stir-fry, bake, boil, or grill your veggies. Just be careful not to cook the life out of them. You can eat the following veggies in their raw form as often as you like:

- Bell peppers
- Celery
- Cucumbers
- Iceberg lettuce
- Parsley
- Radishes
- Romaine lettuce
- Turnips
- Watercress

Other veggies vying for your attention include

- **Garlic and onions:** These veggies are of special interest to
  hypoglycemics and diabetics because they contain special
  sugar-regulating factors. They also reduce LDL ("bad") cholesterol and lower blood pressure. See *Controlling Cholesterol For
  Dummies,* by Carol Ann Rinzler (Wiley), for more info on managing your cholesterol.

- **Artichokes and string beans:** These vegetables are excellent
  for both the hypoglycemic and the diabetic. Artichokes
  improve blood circulation and mobilize energy reserves.
  However, they contain 10 to 14 percent carbs, so eat about a
  quarter of a whole artichoke, and never more than one a day.
  String beans contain an insulin-like hormone and work as a
  sugar balancer.

- **Sprouts and sea vegetables:** Sprouts make good convenience
  foods, because they're easy to grow and inexpensive, and you
  can throw them in many dishes, such as soups and salads, to
  suit your taste. If you want to grow sprouts, you can buy the
  seeds at health food stores. You can use kelp in soups or for
  making stock, and sheets of seaweeds (like the sheets of nori
  that sushi rolls are wrapped in) are handy, versatile, and rich
  in trace minerals. Make sure that you buy unsweetened seaweeds. They're available in most health food stores and Asian
  markets.

Make sure you get enough veggies

Remember that a good minimum is eight servings of veggies daily. However, the ideal amount is anywhere from 10 to 15 servings. Some veggie-happy experts even recommend that for every 50 pounds of body weight, you should eat a pound of raw veggies. (Check out the "Building a hypoglycemic pyramid" section earlier for more specifics.)

How can anyone get such a high proportion of vegetables into their daily diet? It's easier than you may think. Try these ideas:

- ✔ Blend your vegetables into smoothies, possibly adding one or two fresh fruits for a scrumptious taste treat.

- ✔ Make juice from your vegetables. You can mix different vegetables or add a fruit or two. (Avoid juicing only fruits because fruit juices are too high in sugar and trigger a too-rapid increase in your blood sugar.)

If your diet consists mainly of wilted lettuce, mashed potatoes, and overcooked or canned vegetables, or if you think ketchup is a vegetable, you're in for a culinary surprise. Try opening your taste buds to a cornucopia of delights with the dark and leafy greens, and the vivid reds, oranges, yellows, and purples. (The brightly colored ones contain more *antioxidants* — substances that protect you from the free radicals that damage cells.)

The squeaky hypoglycemic gets the grease: Fats

Fats have gotten an undeservedly bad rap in recent years. Too much of the wrong kind of fats is bad, but you do need fats. Your brain is, after all, approximately 70 percent fat. (So if someone calls you a fathead, he's merely stating the truth!) Without fats, you suffer from nerve damage and decreased brain function, not to mention other afflictions, such as hormonal abnormalities and cardiovascular disease. Two fats you should know about are

- ✔ **Saturated fats:** These "bad" fats are found in red meat and high-fat dairy products. You do need some saturated fats, but not very much.

- ✔ **Unsaturated fats:** These "good" fats are found in things like nuts.

The following sections detail which fats you do need and which ones you don't.

Fats you need

In order to function properly, the body needs *essential fatty acids* (EFAs). They're *essential* because they have to come from outside sources — the body can't manufacture them. The long-chain Omega-3 fats from fish and fish oil are particularly beneficial, but they're woefully deficient in the modern diet. Cold-water fish, such as salmon, trout, tuna, and sardines, provide abundant sources of Omega-3 fats. You can also get them from flaxseed oil, chopped walnuts, or eggs that have been enriched with Omega-3. However, fish oil can favorably change the metabolism of fats and carbohydrates — a definite advantage for hypoglycemics who don't tolerate carbs very well.

Although fish is an excellent source of Omega-3 and full of important nutrients, today's fish supply is often contaminated with mercury. This contamination means that larger, predatory fish such as swordfish and shark have unacceptably high levels of mercury. Pregnant women and children younger than 6 should avoid fish altogether. Precaution is recommended for everyone else. A free, online calculator (`www.gotmercury.org`) lets you see which particular seafood is safe to eat.

The best way to get good fats is to drizzle flaxseed oil on your salads, eat fatty, cold-water fish like salmon, and eat avocados (in moderation if you're trying to lose weight). Don't worry about getting too much fat if you're eating lean meats and limiting your consumption of dairy products. The excess fat in most people's diets comes from junk food.

If you're cooking, the best oil to use is coconut oil because high temperatures don't damage it. Coconut oil is a saturated fat that's coming back into favor after many years. Some naturopathic medical doctors recommend coconut oil as particularly beneficial to hypoglycemics because it has a normalizing effect on blood sugar.

Fats you don't

Although too much saturated fat may be bad, trans fatty acids (*trans fat* for short) and altered vegetable fats are extremely destructive and should be avoided. Trans fats have been dubbed *metabolic poison* because they not only elevate your total and LDL ("bad") cholesterol level, but also lower HDL ("good") cholesterol.

Trans fatty acids are artificial fatty acids that block the natural fatty acids. Margarine and many processed snack foods like cakes, cookies, and fries contain these trans fats. (Read the labels and stay away from them.)

Powering up with proteins

Eat some protein at every meal. It ensures slow sugar absorption and helps prevent hypoglycemic symptoms. We're not talking about a huge amount of protein; just a regular, consistent intake to help balance your blood sugar. For a balanced diet, make sure that you obtain your protein from different sources instead of confining yourself to a handful of items that show up in different guises.

The preferred protein sources for hypoglycemics are

- Nuts (macadamia, hazelnut, walnut)
- Seeds (flax, sesame, pumpkin)
- Nut butter (also Tahini and sesame butter)
- Eggs (from free-range chickens)
- Fish and seafood
- Chicken (with the skin removed)
- Turkey (with the skin removed)
- Game meats (rabbit, venison, buffalo, game birds)
- Organ meats (chicken and beef liver)
- Lean meats (organic meats; occasionally pork, if at all)

Meat in the middle (of your whole-wheat bread)

Organic meat comes from livestock raised without hormones and antibiotics. Antibiotics can precipitate hypoglycemia, and hormones may have adverse effects on your health and are better avoided. Try to find meat from grass-fed livestock; it's richer in Omega-3.

You can find organic and grass-fed meat at health food stores. If you can't find any health food stores near your home, check out the sidebar "Using the Web to help you eat healthy" in this chapter. (Of course, if you buy organic meat, you can't just cook it any way you want. Deep frying it or coating it with white flour won't do your hypoglycemia much good.)

Whaddaya, nuts?

Nuts and seeds provide high-quality protein in addition to minerals, fiber, and vitamins E and B-complex, which protect against stress and are involved in mechanisms for blood sugar control. (Chapter 7 has more on minerals and vitamins.)

Perhaps you're afraid to eat nuts because you're concerned about weight. If so, the results of a study of a large group of Americans should put your mind at rest. The study showed that the people who ate the most nuts tended to be less obese (probably because the high amounts of fat and protein in nuts produce a feeling of fullness). Of course, no one is suggesting that eating as many nuts as you want all day long is going to lead to weight reduction!

You can eat two to three servings of nuts per day. One serving is roughly ten whole almonds or peanuts, six walnuts, or two pecans. One serving of seeds is about one tablespoon. Choose nuts without cracks, stains, or splits. Try to purchase them unshelled, raw, and unsalted. If you have to get them shelled, buy whole nuts (not crushed or slivered). Keep them in the fridge and eat them fresh.

Doing dairy

Don't consume more than two to three servings of dairy per day. Eliminate it completely if your hypoglycemic symptoms are severe. Livestock are given antibiotics, which get into the dairy products and encourage the growth of yeasts and fungi that can precipitate allergies, sugar cravings, and hypoglycemia. You can resume eating modest amounts of dairy products after your condition has stabilized. Good sources of dairy are plain, unsweetened whole milk, full-fat yogurt, and raw, organic cheeses.

Breaking the proverbial camel's back: Breads and grains

Carbohydrates are of great interest to hypoglycemics — and diabetics — because they bear the greatest impact on blood sugar levels. Eating the right kinds of carbs in the right amounts is critical in blood sugar management.

Classifying carbs

Carbohydrates can be either simple or complex.

- **Simple carbs** — such as sugar, refined flour, and white rice — are essentially sugars, and they spike your blood sugar rapidly. Simply put, simple carbs are the worst foods for blood sugar control. They're quick burning fuel that skyrockets your blood sugar, only to let it crash, leaving you with low energy and a craving for more sugar and simple carbs. That's why sugars fall into the ugly category of foods that do more harm than good.

The simple avoidance of simple carbs lessens the immediate impact of hypoglycemic symptoms, but to enjoy long-term, radiant good health, your body must obtain the proper nutrients. In short, there is no substitute for wholesome foods.

✔ **Complex carbs** take longer for the body to break down into glucose, and therefore they deliver sugar steadily, making it more likely that blood sugar is stabilized. For the hypoglycemic, this point can't be overemphasized. Whole grains and legumes are slow carbs that release glucose at a slower rate and let you down a little more gently. One caveat: Even complex carbs cause problems if you consume too much.

Whole grains and legumes are complex carbohydrates. Refined grains have their germ and bran removed, which partially or totally eliminates at least 36 nutrients. Whole grains, by contrast, retain these nutrients.

Sticking to complex carbs

Because carbs have a profound effect on your blood sugar level, choose your carbs as wisely as you choose your friends. Whenever possible, choose complex carbs over simple carbs, and choose fruits and vegetables over grains.

Whole grains include the following:

✔ Amaranth

✔ Brown rice

✔ Buckwheat

✔ Quinoa

✔ Unhulled millet

✔ Unpearled barley

✔ Whole oats

✔ Whole wheat

Legumes provide two to four times as much protein as grains. They also help improve liver function and blood sugar control. They include

✔ Black eyed peas

✔ Chickpeas

✔ Garbanzo beans

✔ Kidney beans

✔ Lentils

✔ Lima beans

✔ Pinto beans

You can find grains and legumes in natural food stores. They're often sold in bulk, so you can easily find the right ones by just looking at the labels — or by asking a store clerk. (If you can't find them in bulk, look for them in packages or cartons with labels.)

Eating the Right Way

Eating right is *the* key to reducing your hypoglycemia symptoms and possibly even eliminating them all together. We wager that you'll be pleasantly surprised at how good you feel after you embark on your recovery program.

This section covers the importance of eating the right way, starting with eating smaller meals, smaller serving sizes, and a healthy breakfast. This section also gives you some helpful pointers that provide just the essential info so you can start eating better.

Starting off on the right foot

The beginning of any program is crucial because it sets the foundation. It can mean the difference between success and failure. For the hypoglycemic in particular, starting right is important because if you do, you'll have the incentive to stay on track because your symptoms are likely to start abating quite quickly.

What to do initially

When you begin your hypoglycemia-eating program, take the following steps to help ensure success:

✔ **Limit fruits to two servings a day.** As your condition improves, you can eat four to five servings a day. (A serving is one small orange or apple.) However, if you have a strong craving for sweets, and you feel like you're going to break down and gorge on forbidden pastries (like chocolate cake), grab a fruit — even if it means exceeding your daily quota.

✔ **Exercise caution with the carbs from bread, cereal, rice, and pasta.** When you begin your dietary program, you can get faster results by completely eliminating this group. After a month or two, you can reintroduce these foods into your diet. Even then, limit them to no more than four servings per day — two servings a day, ideally. If you start experiencing hypoglycemic symptoms, cut back immediately.

✔ **Eat mostly raw foods.** Gradually add more raw vegetables and fruit to your diet until you're consuming about one-third of your foods raw. Doing so ensures that you're getting enzymes and essential micronutrients that cooking destroys.

✔ **Consume more vegetables.** Vegetables should be a regular part of each meal. (Check out "Eating the best veggies in the best state [raw, that is]" earlier in this chapter.) However, be careful about which vegetables you eat. In the initial phase of your recovery, eliminate potatoes and cut back on root vegetables that grow underground because they have a high amount of starch.

✔ **Drink enough water.** How much depends on various factors such as your weight, your health, how active you are, and where you live. The more active you are, the more fluid you need. You also need to drink more if you live in hot, humid climates, or if you're running a fever. In general, drink between 9 to 13 cups of water a day. If you rarely feel thirsty, and your urine is colorless or slightly yellow, you're probably drinking enough.

✔ **Maintain a regular sleep and wake schedule seven days a week.** Nothing sabotages your progress faster than lack of sleep. Sleep deprivation can make you reach for a candy bar or something equally sugary. When you have low blood sugar at night, it keeps you from sleeping well and gives you nightmares. To avoid such a scenario, eat a bit of protein before you go to bed, but make sure it's a very small portion that doesn't promote weight gain. (Taking magnesium supplements can also help promote sound sleep and help prevent diabetes.)

As a general rule, aim for at least 30 percent protein and 30 percent fat early in your program. As you progress in your recovery, cut back on protein and increase your consumption of carbs. Do so gradually, noting any reappearance of symptoms.

Touching base: How are you doing?

If you stick to your food plan, by the end of the third or fourth month, you should be generally clear of most hypoglycemic symptoms, although a more complete recovery may take six months or longer. For some individuals, the improvements start within the first month, or as early as the first couple of weeks. (Again, bear in mind the individual differences among people.) When you're clear of most of your symptoms, you should be eating 25 percent protein, 50 percent carbs, and 25 percent good fats. One-third to one-half of the fats in each meal should be in the form of essential fatty acids, and you should have 35 to 45 grams of dietary fiber a day.

Dr. Colleen Huber, a naturopath with extensive experience treating hypoglycemics, believes that some symptoms of hypoglycemia may, in fact, be caused by the lack of fiber in the diet. Therefore, incorporate fiber into your diet. You may start out on the higher end of the fat and protein consumption guidelines when you embark on the program for recovery and then gradually begin cutting back.

 This dietary plan is for hypoglycemics. Diabetics can generally eat diets designed for hypoglycemics. However, if you're diabetic, you *must* be vigilant about serving sizes and food exchanges. For more information, see *Diabetes Cookbook For Dummies,* by Alan L. Rubin, MD (Wiley).

Eating six meals — or more — a day

The good news is that being hypoglycemic means never having to say you're hungry. That's because you get to eat three small meals and three snacks (or six small meals if you prefer) at two to three hour intervals. Some individuals may need to eat even more frequently, eight or more times a day. (See the nearby sidebar, "Snacking it up," if you need ideas for healthy snacks.)

 Start out with six meals a day, and gauge how you feel. Do you feel shaky and hungry? Then eat more often. Time yourself to work out what best suits your needs. The object is to ensure that your blood sugar never drops too low. Even if you don't have much of an appetite, you shouldn't let too many hours go without eating — except when you're sleeping. But remember to make your meals and snacks correspondingly smaller (or lower in calories), or you'll end up gaining weight!

The most important meal

 A blood-sugar balanced day begins with a good breakfast. Don't omit eating a good breakfast if you suffer from hypoglycemia. You want to eat either immediately or shortly after you wake up, preferably within an hour, and definitely not longer than two hours. (For more on the dilemma, check out the sidebar, "Darned if you do, darned if you donut" in this chapter.)

Breakfast seems to have the biggest impact on blood sugar. In addition, eating the right foods for breakfast sets the tone for the rest of the day. Some good foods include plain, unsweetened, whole-fat yogurt, a hard-boiled egg, or oatmeal cooked with an egg. Stay away from traditional breakfast foods such as bacon, pancakes, donuts, or bagels.

If you're in the habit of exercising and/or meditating for more than an hour before breakfast, take some protein powder before your workout to prevent a blood sugar drop. If you don't, you may be tempted to gobble down anything that gives you instant energy. (*Protein powder* is a concentrated form of protein that you can drink like a shake. Read labels to make sure that the protein powder you choose doesn't have any added sugars. You can get powdered whey protein, soy protein, or an alternative vegetarian protein powder at health food stores or on the Internet.)

Don't feel like having breakfast? Then at least eat a small amount of food, like a few tablespoons of plain, whole-fat yogurt immediately after waking up.

Sizing up your servings

When you're sticking to a healthy diet, you need to watch your serving sizes (for info on what you should eat, see "Of Food Pyramids and Healthy Eating," earlier in this chapter). You're ahead of the game if you're familiar with serving sizes. Fear not if you haven't a clue what a serving platter is (much less a serving size).

You don't have to measure your foods precisely: You're not conducting a chemical experiment! You probably won't be able to stick with a diet that requires you to accurately weigh or measure everything you eat. Besides, you'd look pretty silly if you pulled out a scale when eating out.

Think of one serving as roughly

- ✔ 1 slice whole grain bread
- ✔ ½ cup oatmeal or other cooked whole grains
- ✔ 1 cup carrots
- ✔ ½ cup beans, peas, or lentils
- ✔ ½ cup corn
- ✔ 1 small apple, orange, or pear
- ✔ 1 medium peach or nectarine
- ✔ ½ banana
- ✔ ½ cup pineapple
- ✔ ¼ melon

To familiarize yourself with a serving size, measure some foods you eat. That way, you'll have a visual estimate of how much you're eating. According to the American Dietetic Association (ADA), most people overestimate serving sizes. Table 6-1 offers the ADA's helpful visual comparisons for estimating one serving size.

Table 6-1	Estimating a Serving Size
Food	*What a Serving Size Looks Like*
Cooked lean meat, poultry, or fish (2–3 ounces)	An audiocassette or personal digital assistant
Cheese (1.5 ounces)	Four stacked dice
Fruit, cooked vegetables, cooked rice or pasta	Tennis ball cut in half
Raw leafy vegetables	Tennis ball

Getting back on the wagon if you've fallen off

What if you've been down this primrose path before, eating six, eight, even eleven times a day, and you're still not finding the relief you want? How can you get back on this diet and stick with it? Remember these simple pointers:

- **Make sure you're eating regularly and not skipping any meals or snacks.** Don't wait until you're hungry to eat.

- **Set up a timer or other reminders.** You can easily get immersed in whatever you're doing and forget to eat at regular intervals.

- **See whether eating even more frequently helps.** Each person is different. Perhaps you need to eat even more often than most people in order to keep your blood sugar on an even keel. The only way to find out is by experimenting.

- **Review your diet to see whether you've really and truly been following the basic hypoglycemia diet.** Have you eliminated all simple carbs? Are you getting enough fiber? Protein? Vegetables? (This is why a food journal is so important; refer to "Chewing on a Food Journal" later in this chapter for more info.)

Snacking it up

Most hypoglycemics benefit from eating every two to three hours. Here are some ideas for snacks:

✔ Nut butter, miso, or hummus spread on celery, cucumber, or other vegetables. Some people enjoy almond butter on apples.

✔ Plain nuts and seeds. These are good alone or combined.

✔ Japanese rice crackers.

✔ Baked apples with a dollop of butter.

✔ Baked sweet potato.

✔ Hot azuki soup sweetened with stevia (simply cook azuki beans in water, and then add stevia).

✔ A small portion of leftovers from a meal.

You may be slipping without even knowing. Be very honest. And remember, your symptoms may persist for awhile. Although every individual is different, you may notice a significant difference in six weeks.

Adding helpful food substitutes

To reduce the intake of carbohydrates — especially that of grains — substitute vegetables for grains. Try the following subs:

✔ **Bread substitutes:** Use greens such as romaine lettuce as wraps. You can also use cabbage, celery, cucumber, and other raw vegetables.

✔ **Rice substitute:** Steam a head of cauliflower until soft and mash it up a bit.

✔ **Soup thickeners:** Powdered kuzu from kuzu root (good as cooking starch; also soothes digestive disorders), arrow root, and potato starch are good options.

✔ **Milk substitutes:** Try rice, almond, and hazelnut milk with no added sweetener. You can also drink soy milk occasionally.

✔ **Wheat flour substitutes for people with wheat allergies:** Try kamut, millet (makes baked goods coarse and dry), barley (may contain some gluten), brown rice (tends to be crumbly), corn, quinoa, amaranth, and spelt. Buckwheat and oat flour may be used for variety, but they do contain some gluten.

When baking, experiment by adding more water. If the mixture is too dry, add an egg. Some flours work well in combination. For instance, kamut can be mixed with spelt.

✔ **Coffee substitutes:** Health food stores carry many delicious grain coffees and other healthy substitutes. (Check out Chapter 11 for more coffee substitutes.)

Hypoglycemia in Vegetarians: What Can You Eat?

So you skip the animal flesh. No eggs or dairy, either? You have to make sure that you get enough protein and avoid eating too many grains and carbohydrates. Hypoglycemics may have a higher protein need in the initial stages of their recovery. Consider trying some of the following to make sure you get enough protein:

✔ **Legumes:** A traditional source of protein is legumes (such as beans and lentils), which were known as "the poor man's meat" in the early part of the 19th century. Be aware, however, that they're much higher in carbohydrates than they are in protein, so they should be supplemented with other protein sources; at the same time, you need to go easy on eating other forms of carbs so that you don't get a carb-overload.

✔ **Fish:** If you're not a strict vegetarian, fish can be an excellent way to complement your diet as long as you eat no more than one serving per week, and you choose varieties that are relatively free of mercury.

✔ **Soy foods:** Foods such as tofu (bean curd) and tempeh (cheese-like cooked beans) are extremely versatile, and you can make literally hundreds of dishes with various forms of soy. No wonder it's the preferred source of protein for many vegetarians, as well as health-conscious meat-eaters. But too much of a good thing can compromise your health. Recent research appears to show that soybeans may be a bit of a mixed bag. Until the final verdict comes in, here's what we recommend:

  • Limit your intake to no more than two to three servings of whole soy foods a day.

  • Avoid eating soy every day of the week.

  • Eat more fermented soy products, such as miso and natto. Fermentation achieves a biochemical transformation that neutralizes the objectionable ingredients in soy.

✔ **Raw seeds:** Eat them with or without nuts.

> ✔ **Algae:** Spirulina and chlorella are also sources of protein. Chlorella in particular regulates blood sugar and helps to reduce the craving for carbs.

Supplement your diet with fish oil capsules or flaxseed oil so that you get enough essential fatty acids (EFAs). Walnuts are also good sources of these EFAs. You may also add an occasional egg or natural cheese. To help end cruelty to animals, look for eggs from *free-range chickens* (ones that aren't cooped up).

Chewing on a Food Journal

Keeping a daily food journal is the backbone of your recovery process and of personalizing the general plan. The object of the food journal is to help you see exactly what you're doing. It helps you become aware of the foods and beverages you're consuming. With a journal, you can start to see the connection between what goes into your mouth and your moods, feelings, and bodily sensations.

Find a notebook that you like and feel comfortable using. You can get a regular notebook, or you can purchase something that's constructed of handmade paper or bound in leather. If you prefer, carry around large index cards or loose paper, and then staple them together at the end of the week. Make sure that you write the date clearly on each card or page. You can also use a micro-cassette recorder; if you do, we still recommend that you transcribe everything onto paper at the end of the day (or several days) so you can reference it later and track your progress.

This section explains what a food journal can do for you and how you can use it to keep focused on your diet.

Knowing what to record

When you keep your daily food journal, make sure that you write down the following things:

> ✔ Exactly what you eat and drink.
>
> ✔ What exercises you engage in (check out Chapter 8).
>
> ✔ Your feelings, both physical and emotional. Rating your feelings on a scale of 1 to 10, from the least to the most intense, may be helpful. (Check out the next section for more info.)

✔ Anything else that seems relevant (you may also want to add comments).

✔ An overall rating for the entire day, again on a scale of 1 to 10. Doing so makes it easier to note any progress or setbacks.

By recording this information, you can make your journal a helpful resource. You journal can also

✔ **Keep you focused and aware of what you're eating and drinking and how you're feeling.** It can help keep you on track. (Check out the section "Tracking your progress" later in this chapter.)

✔ **Prevent you from engaging your mental autopilot and consuming foods unconsciously.** If you park yourself in front of the TV, it's very easy to eat a bag of chips or guzzle down an entire six-pack without really being aware of what you're doing.

✔ **Help you keep track of food-related symptoms and identify any food sensitivities you have.** When you experience any symptoms, go back to your food journal and see what foods you've eaten just before the symptoms started. You should also track foods down as far back as 24 to 48 hours — sometimes maybe even longer. Over time, you can detect a pattern.

✔ **Help you pay attention to yourself.** It may even be the first time in your adult life that you've taken the time to do so. As you continue to write in your journal, you'll begin to discover your own needs and rhythms. You may be so accustomed to taking your cues from others outside of yourself — your parents, your peers, television commercials — that perhaps you've forgotten how to listen to your own body.

Don't worry if you forget to write things down, or if you don't know how to explain your feelings. Gradually, you'll become adept at recognizing your feelings. It's important to accept whatever you're feeling without blaming or criticizing yourself.

A food journal isn't just for food

Write down any physical or emotional changes you may be experiencing. For instance, if you have more energy or you're unusually irritable, be sure to note it. Instead of jotting down your feelings only after you eat, make a point of writing them down every hour or two. Recording your feelings can make it easier to see how certain foods (or combinations of foods) affect your mood or physical symptoms. You don't have to write lengthy essays — just a word or two will suffice.

When you write what you're feeling on a regular basis, you may begin to uncover

- ✔ Connections between foods that you never suspected before
- ✔ Whether a recurrent feeling is triggered by something you eat or by the stresses in your life
- ✔ What's working or not working in terms of your diet
- ✔ Where and how you drifted from your eating program (if you did drift; what are you, superhuman?)

The more you know about what's going on with yourself, the easier it is to make any necessary adjustments in your life. Highlight your journal, and circle any links you see. Have fun while becoming your own private investigator.

Tracking your progress

Look over your journal every week. If you can, look it over on the same day of the week (Sunday, for example) so that you don't forget. After you start identifying the patterns and feeling more confident about your food choices (perhaps in a month or two), you can review every two weeks. But if you notice anything unusual (like the appearance of certain symptoms), don't wait to refer to your journal.

If keeping a food journal seems too overwhelming for you right now, don't get discouraged. When you have chronic low blood sugar, getting focused or motivated is hard. Just do the best you can. It all starts coming together when you start feeling better. Until then, try jotting any unusual symptoms or anything else of note on your calendar. At the end of the day, give a numerical rating to the day. This method may give you the momentum and motivation to try the more complete version of the food diary.

Keeping a daily food journal helps you make refinements and get better results. On the other hand, avoid straying too far from the basic recommendations. You'll know when you aren't following your diet correctly, because your hypoglycemic symptoms (see Chapter 3 if you need a refresher on symptoms) will reappear. Don't sweat it if they do; just get right back to following your healthy eating plan.

Chapter 7

Hanging with Herb and His Buddies Vitamin and Supplement

Should you take vitamin and mineral supplements? The next time you're bored in a meeting, bring up this question. Add to the discussion a disorder that some people argue doesn't even exist, and there you have a fine debate.

Although dietary therapy is the cornerstone of hypoglycemia treatment, anyone suffering from blood sugar imbalance has an increased need for many nutrients that aren't easy to obtain only from food. Nutritional supplements handle many symptoms as well as help improve blood sugar control.

This chapter shows you how to use herbs, vitamins, and minerals to address specific hypoglycemic symptoms and discomforts. Chapters 8, 9, and 10 show you additional ways you can cope and survive — even thrive — with this metabolic disorder.

Getting Acquainted with Herb

When you get to know "Herb," you find that he's a pretty interesting fellow. He's been around for a long time, all over the world. Yes, herbs have probably been used since the dawn of humankind, and herbal medicine is no passing fad. Traditionally, people in Europe, India, and China have relied on herbal medicine to prevent and heal illnesses.

Humans treat a variety of complaints — from insomnia to allergies — with herbal remedies. In some cases, *herbs* (roots, flowers, and other parts of plants with medicinal properties) can be just as (or more) effective in treating common ailments as prescription and over-the-counter medications; they're generally safer, too.

This effectiveness in treating ailments doesn't mean, however, that herbs are completely safe. Being natural doesn't mean that something is completely without side effects — some substances can be "naturally poisonous," after all. Also, before combining herbal treatments with prescription medications, check with your physician and an experienced herbal practitioner.

As long as you use herbs as instructed and take them in the right doses, they have a good safety record. Some herbalists warn that certain herbs or formulas taken for a long time can lead to toxicity. So don't continue to take something for longer than you need it, and take breaks from the products. Keep in mind that these are just general guidelines; everyone reacts to herbs differently. What works for your Aunt Ninny may not work for you.

Saying Hello to Supplements and Vitamins

Not only did Mom tell you to eat your veggies, but she also made you down those nasty-tasting vitamins. Who knew she was right? And do you know what *supplements* really are? They're nutrients, such as vitamins and minerals, that you add to your regular diet in the form of pills, powders, or liquids. This section takes a closer look at what vitamins, minerals, and supplements are and their roles in a balanced diet.

Vitamins and minerals

Vitamins, which are vital to the regulation of *metabolic processes* (chemical changes in living cells by which energy is provided) are generally classified as being one of the following:

- ✔ **Water soluble:** These aren't stored in the body. Any excess gets flushed into the urine — for this reason, some doctors insist that all you get from taking vitamins is expensive urine.

✔ **Fat soluble:** This type is stored in the body, so be careful not to take too much. These vitamins can build up to a toxic level. The fat-soluble vitamins are A, D, E, and K. Some doctors discourage supplementation, because they're afraid that people will be careless and take too much. This isn't usually a problem, unless you're taking megadoses for an extended period of time.

The American Medical Association and the National Academy of Sciences continue to maintain their official stance by saying that supplementation has no benefits as long as you're eating a proper, well-balanced diet. Yet a large and growing body of evidence suggests that you can gain significant health benefits from taking vitamins. Many medical doctors are beginning to recognize that vitamins and minerals, often in amounts that are difficult to get through food alone, can alleviate certain conditions.

If you take a daily vitamin, we recommend giving your body a break from the vitamin pill, because your body can become habituated to it, decreasing its effectiveness. By stopping from time to time, you'll still enjoy the benefits of supplementation while reducing the costs. Take vitamins for one month straight and then go off them for a week. Or you can take them for six days and break for one day. For more information on vitamins, see *Vitamins For Dummies,* by Christopher Hobbs, LAc, and Elson Haas, MD (Wiley).

Supplements

Nutritional *supplements* are vitamins in the form of tablets, capsules, powders, or liquids, and they can be natural or synthetic. *Natural vitamins* are derived from natural sources — from plant or animal tissues — while *synthetic vitamins* are created artificially to assume the same chemical structure as the natural vitamin.

Choose natural vitamins whenever you can, because they may contain substances that scientists aren't necessarily aware of yet that may provide extra benefits. Besides, the substances found in natural vitamins remain in their natural ratio, which works better. Synthetic vitamins may also have added artificial colorings and flavorings that you're better off without. Always read the labels to make sure that your vitamins contain no added sugar, yeast, or preservatives. The label tells you whether the vitamin is natural or synthetic.

Never let taking supplements be an excuse for eating poorly. Aim to get as many nutrients as possible from actual foods.

Taking the Hypoglycemia Mix

Table 7-1 shows the basic list of daily vitamins that nutritionists and practitioners have found to be beneficial to people suffering from hypoglycemia. Please note that the dosages listed in the table are meant only as general guidelines. The recommended dosage levels vary with a patient's age, activity level, and current nutritional status. You can easily get the recommended levels by taking a good multiple vitamin and mineral formula (for resources on where to buy them, see the sidebar, "Jumping on the Net for more alternatives") and then adding specific nutrients that may be missing or that aren't provided in high enough amounts. (*Note:* Multiple vitamin and mineral formulas sold at supermarkets and drug stores are generally not the best kind.)

Although they're higher than the Recommended Daily Allowance (RDA), the following dosages aren't considered megadoses, and taking them shouldn't result in any unwanted side effects. However, consult your primary care physician before you begin.

All the ingredients in supplements should appear on the label. The amounts in Table 7-1 are given in milligrams (mg), micrograms (mcg), and international units (IU). These measurements are different ways of expressing the amount of vitamins and minerals in a tablet or capsule. A milligram is $\frac{1}{1000}$ of a gram, while a microgram is $\frac{1}{1000}$ of a milligram. IU is an international standard of measurement for vitamins A, D, and E. There's no fixed definition for IU; it's different for each substance.

Table 7-1:   Vitamins and Minerals that Can Benefit Hypoglycemics if Taken Daily

Vitamin	Amount Per Day	Benefit
Vitamin A (acetate)	5,000 IU	Maintains healthy skin and good eyesight; treats acute infections.
Vitamin A (beta carotene)	10,000 IU	A double-vitamin A molecule that the body can eliminate, and therefore unlike vitamin A acetate doesn't accumulate and cause toxicity.
Vitamin C	2,000 mg	Supports the adrenal glands.

Vitamin	Amount Per Day	Benefit
Vitamin D	200 IU	Helps the body absorb and use calcium.
Vitamin E (d-alpha tocopheryl acetate)	400 IU	Prevents degenerative diseases of the cardiovascular, neurological, and respiratory systems.
Thiamine (Vitamin B1)	100 mg	Converts glucose to energy and is important for adrenal glands. Crucial for a healthy nervous system.
Riboflavin (Vitamin B2)	50–100 mg	Helps regulate mood. Crucial for a healthy nervous system.
Niacin (Vitamin B3)	100 mg	Converts glucose to energy and is important for adrenal glands. Crucial for a healthy nervous system.
Niacinamide (Vitamin B3)	50–75 mg	Helps metabolize carbs, fats, and proteins, as well as reduce high cholesterol levels and plays a role in removing toxic and harmful chemicals from the body.
Pantothenic acid (Vitamin B5)	1,000 mg	Aids adrenal function and plays an important role in the production of energy.
Pyridoxine (Vitamin B6)	50 mg	Metabolizes protein and is crucial in the proper functioning of the nervous and immune systems. Deficiencies in Vitamin B6 are sometimes linked to hypoglycemia.
Vitamin B12	400–1,000 mcg	Converts glucose to energy and is important for adrenal glands. Crucial for a healthy nervous system.
Biotin	300 mcg	Plays an essential role in the production of fatty and amino acids. Important in food metabolism.
Folic acid	400–1,000 mcg	Helps reduce heart and cardiovascular diseases and can help prevent birth defects.

(continued)

Table 7-1 *(continued)*

Mineral	Amount Per Day	Benefit
Boron	1–2 mg	Helps the bones use calcium. May also help regulate calcium, magnesium, and phosphorous balance.
Calcium	1,500 mg	Metabolizes sugar.
Chromium	400 mcg	Metabolizes carbohydrates and is essential for insulin function.
Copper	1 mg	Helps in the healthy functioning of nerves and joints.
Iodine	75 mcg	Helps the thyroid control metabolic rate and body temperature.
Magnesium	750 mg	Helps metabolize sugar.
Manganese	10 mg	Helps the body utilize vitamin C and some B vitamins; facilitates glucose metabolism.
Molybdenum	50 mcg	Helps metabolize carbohydrates.
Potassium	200 mg	Supports electrical impulses across cell membranes. Assists in body's energy use.
Selenium	200 mcg	Functions as part of the body's detoxifying systems. Important in cancer prevention.
Zinc	50 mg	Plays crucial role in glucose and insulin regulation.

Some vitamins and minerals should be taken in *divided doses,* so you don't take the entire dose at once. In other words, if you're taking 1,500 mg of calcium a day, you can take 500 mg in the morning, 500 at noon, and 500 in the evening. Take these vitamins in divided doses for better overall absorption:

- ✓ Calcium
- ✓ Magnesium
- ✓ Vitamin C
- ✓ Thiamin

   ✔ Niacin

   ✔ Vitamin B12

   ✔ Pantothenic acid

In addition to taking the previously mentioned vitamins and minerals daily, you may want to include the supplements described in Table 7-2. They're particularly helpful because they support glucose and insulin metabolism, facilitate glands involved in blood-sugar regulation, raise blood sugar levels, and/or enhance mood.

Table 7-2: Additional Supplements that Can Benefit Hypoglycemics if Taken Daily

Supplement	Amount Per Day	Benefit
L-glutamine. Do *not* take if you have Reye's syndrome, cirrhosis of the liver, or kidney problems.	1 gram on an empty stomach	This amino acid (which is most abundant in the body) raises blood sugar levels and reduces fatigue. Also energizes the brain and maintains a healthy digestive system.
L-tyrosine. Consult your doctor before taking if you have lupus. Do *not* use if you're taking MAO inhibitors.	1–2 grams	This amino acid enhances mood and facilitates adrenal, thyroid, and pituitary functioning.
CLA (Conjugated linolenic acid)	3,000–4,000 mg	This natural fatty acid supports the healthy metabolism of glucose and insulin.

If you're on a very tight budget that doesn't allow for vitamins, then you're going to have to be more stringent and careful with your diet. Put all your available resources for healing into high-quality foods. (Flip to Chapter 6 for complete instructions.) Perhaps you're in a tight spot financially because of your battle with hypoglycemia. After you stabilize your blood sugar, you may find your entire life — including your finances — changing for the better. Begin taking all the recommended vitamins and supplements then, when you have the financial means to do so without breaking the bank.

Jumping on the Net for more alternatives

We provide tons of helpful info in this chapter if you're seriously considering taking vitamins, herbs, and supplements to counter your hypoglycemia. If you want even more info, check out the following Web sites:

✔ **American Botanical Council (www.herbalgram.org):** This council provides science-based information that promotes the safe use of herbal medicines. The Web site has information on herbs, a list of resources, and critical reviews of current journal articles.

✔ **Dr. Murray Natural Living (www.doctormurray.com):** Dr. Murray is the author of nearly 30 books on health-related topics and offers nutritional guidance on health conditions through this site. Readers can ask him questions and access articles, lectures, and newsletters. The site sells nutritional supplements, including a special formula for hypoglycemics.

✔ **Good Cause Wellness (www.goodcausewellness.com/servlet/StoreFront):** This site offers various nutritional supplements and blended fruits and vegetables. It also sells chia seeds, which are very high in Omega-3 fatty acids, and a granola mix of goji, blueberry, and chia seeds.

✔ **Herbal Advantage, Inc. (www.herbaladvantage.com):** Herbal Advantage, Inc., sells stevia and other herbs, spices, and natural items.

✔ **Naturopathy Works (www.naturopathyworks.com):** The Web site of Naturopathic Medical Doctor Colleen Huber features free newsletters and articles on botanicals, Chinese medicine, environmental medicine, homeopathy, nutrition, physical medicine, and hydrotherapy. The site has a table showing cravings for unhealthy foods, such as sweets and oily foods, and the nutrient deficiencies that are behind these cravings. Also listed are healthy foods rich in the missing nutrients.

✔ **Nordic Naturals (www.nordicnaturals.com):** This site sells supplements for humans and pets, and specializes in Omega-3 and Omega-6 essential fatty acids and cod liver oil.

✔ **Nutribiotic (hono.stores.yahoo.net/nutribiotic.html):** This is a complete online vitamin and supplement source. Products include rice protein powder, nutrition bars, low-carb products, flower essences, and beauty products.

✔ **Nutrition Dynamics (www.nutritiondynamics.com):** This Web site sells herbs, supplements, enzymes, and homeopathic remedies; it also offers detailed information on vitamins.

✔ **Pain Net (www.painnet.com):** This Web site provides information about pain management, sources for information about pain and its causes, newsletters, listings for pain medicine practitioners in each state, a link to online counseling, and a bookstore.

✔ **Thorne Research, Inc. (www.thorne.com):** This Web site offers high-quality nutritional supplements, an alternative medicine review, and a quarterly newsletter.

If you do have any extras leftover for spending, get the following supplements, because they're likely to have the most direct impact on stabilizing blood sugar and keeping your symptoms at bay:

- **Chromium (GTF):** Take a minimum of 200–500 micrograms in the form of chromium picolinate per day. Some nutritionists recommend at least 600 mcg daily or even as much as 1,000 mcg daily. If you find yourself frequently craving sugar, you may have a low level of chromium in your body.

- **The amino acid 5-Hydroxytryptophan (5-HTP):** It's said to be effective for carbohydrate cravings. Take 50–100 mg three times a day. 5-HTP is also the direct precursor to *serotonin,* the neurotransmitter that plays a critical role in the regulation of mood. It can be helpful for some people in the treatment of depression. 5-HTP loses its effectiveness if taken continuously, so refrain from taking it for one to two days each week.

- **Omega-3 essential fatty acid:** Take a minimum of 3,000 mg daily, in the form of fish oil liquid or capsules. Omega-3s are essential, but the body can't make them — you must get them through food. Unfortunately, the modern diet is woefully deficient in Omega-3. Getting a supplement is important for people with blood sugar problems because the amount of Omega-3 you get is directly related to how sensitive the cells are to insulin, the key hormone in balancing blood sugar.

  Studies suggest that Omega-3 supplementation may help with depression, aggression, eczema, attention deficit disorder (ADD), and blood pressure.

  Some nutritionists recommend that patients who want to improve their carbohydrate metabolism should initially saturate their system by taking a total of 6,000 mg Omega-3 daily.

 Make sure that any product you're taking is pure and processed properly. For example, mercury and lead are common contaminants in fish oil. If your product is tainted, the supplement will damage rather than improve your health.

Matching Supplements to Ails: Which Makes You Feel Better?

This section gets to the fun part: symptoms! Fortunately, you can summon stalwart supporters to your aid. We list some of the most common symptoms of hypoglycemia and things you can take to alleviate them.

You're not going to have all the symptoms listed in the following sections, and even though the symptoms are associated with hypoglycemia, having one or more of them and *not* having the disorder is possible. If you want to know more about the symptoms of hypoglycemia, flip to Chapter 3.

See your primary care physician before starting a supplemental program. In addition, when you consult with any healthcare practitioner, always let her know exactly what supplements you're taking.

Anxiety

Are you anxious about everything? Are you just plain anxious about nothing in particular? People are more prone to feeling aches and pains when they're suffering from anxiety.

Some supplements are good for helping control anxiety. They can be too stimulating, making it hard for you to sleep, so be careful not to take the following supplements at night:

- ✔ **GABA (gamma-amino butyric acid):** You can find this amino acid and neurotransmitter in capsule form. Take the recommended dosage described on the product.

- ✔ **Inositol:** This vitamin-like substance is often grouped with the B vitamins. A study showed that its effects are similar to those of mild tranquilizers. *Therapeutic doses* (amounts high enough to have a medicinal effect on the person taking it) of inositol range from 500–1,000 mg per day. In some sensitive individuals, too high a dose can cause diarrhea.

- ✔ **Kava kava:** This herb can help you relax but remain alert. Kava kava contains active ingredients that are thought to work like aspirin. Look for it in *tinctures* (highly concentrated liquid herbal extracts) and capsules at herbal shops.

  Some studies have linked it with severe liver damage. Although such cases are rare, the potential risk exists. Take the herb only under the guidance of a qualified healthcare practitioner. Furthermore, pregnant or nursing women are strongly advised against taking it. Also, be aware that if you take alcohol or barbiturates, kava kava will have a stronger effect on you.

- ✔ **Passionflower:** This herb is especially effective if you have anxiety attacks in the middle of the night. You can brew passionflower into a tea (steep two teaspoons of the dried herb for 30 minutes in a cup of freshly boiled water), or you can consume it in a tincture. Don't use it for more than two weeks.

✔ **Skullcap:** This herb, which contains minerals such as calcium, iron, potassium, and magnesium, revitalizes the nervous system. It eases stress, anxiety, and depression, as well as alleviates premenstrual syndrome. Use as an extract.

✔ **Vitamin B:** Make sure that you're getting enough of this vitamin. Studies on both humans and animals suggest an association between anxiety and deficiencies of vitamin B complex. Take 25–100 mg of vitamin B complex a day, as a single dose or in *divided doses* (the required dose split into two or three doses).

If you have recurrent, long-standing anxiety problems that aren't caused by medical conditions, you should definitely make meditation, deep breathing, and relaxation exercises a part of your daily life. (Chapter 9 can help.) Because anxiety and depression often go hand in hand, you may want to refer to the sections "Depression/mood swings" and "Stress," later in this chapter.

Asthma

People who suffer from asthma have labored breathing often accompanied by wheezing, coughing, or gasping. They may experience a sense of constriction in the chest.

The following supplements can help reduce the severity of asthma attacks; you shouldn't, however, under any circumstances, substitute these remedies for what your doctor prescribes you. In case of a serious attack, call your doctor or go to the emergency room.

✔ **Fish oil capsules:** The oil should be from fish high in anti-inflammatory Omega-3 fatty acids (salmon, mackerel, sardines, and tuna). You have to take these capsules for ten weeks or so before you start noticing benefits.

Avoid fish oils if you're allergic to fish.

✔ **Garlic:** Garlic works as a mucus regulator for chronic bronchitis. Garlic cooked with chicken soup is especially nourishing. Inhaling the fumes while the soup is cooking can help alleviate symptoms. Sip the soup throughout the day.

✔ **Nettle:** Nettle (in the form of root juice or leaves) can help relieve asthma symptoms and allergies. Some very potent ginger extracts naturally reduce inflammation throughout the body.

✔ **Turmeric:** This Indian spice is a good anti-inflammatory. The whole spice, however, isn't potent enough. Instead, get capsules with curcumin, and take at least 400 mg daily.

Chronic fatigue syndrome

If you have hypoglycemia associated with chronic fatigue syndrome, the following supplements may provide some relief:

- **Ashwaganda root:** It energizes by nourishing the kidneys.

- **Astragalus:** It strengthens the immune system by helping the body produce antibodies and working in the bone marrow to produce white blood cells.

- **DHEA (dehydroepiandrosterone):** DHEA improves neurological function, immune function, and stress disorders. Women shouldn't exceed 15mg per day, and men shouldn't exceed 25mg per day, unless blood levels are monitored by a physician or other health professional.

- **Echinacea:** Good for fighting colds, flu, and infections, echinacea boosts the immune system.

- **Ginkgo biloba:** It improves circulation, sharpens memory, reduces anxiety, and boosts concentration.

- **Hydrocortisone:** Used in the treatment of chronically stressed and weakened adrenals.

- **Licorice:** No, not the candy! Don't take this supplement if you have high blood pressure. Licorice has anti-inflammatory, anti-allergic, and anti-arthritic properties.

- **NADH (nicotinamide adenine dinucleotide):** It's found in all living cells, and it's essential for their development and energy production. Helps fight fatigue.

- **SAM-e (S-adenosyl-methionine):** It's an amino acid derivative that's normally synthesized in the body. Some evidence suggests that it may be a fast-acting, safe, and effective antidepressant.

- **Siberian ginseng:** Useful in fighting stress and fatigue, Siberian ginseng protects the liver and helps prevent memory loss and boosts energy.

Constipation

Who hasn't suffered from constipation at one time or another? Thanks to the modern diet, it's become a common problem in the so-called civilized world. Just staying away from sugar and refined flour should soon relieve (indeed!) your problem. The following remedies may help relieve constipation:

✔ **Allicin:** This substance found in garlic stimulates the contractions of the intestinal walls. Eating garlic by itself can upset your stomach, so you may want to stir-fry it with onions or mix it with yogurt to help buffer it.

✔ **Radishes:** Yes, that reddish root vegetable can help alleviate constipation, too. Radishes in yogurt may be interesting, but they'll probably taste better in a salad.

✔ **Whole grain barley:** Try eating whole grain barley products (the less processed, the better).

If you have chronic problems with constipation, or if you haven't produced a BM for a week or longer, see your doctor.

Depression/mood swings

After you stabilize your blood sugar, your depression should begin to ease (unless underlying problems exist). If you're hypoglycemic, make sure that you follow the recommended dietary changes in this book or the changes outlined by your healthcare practitioner. That alone should make a significant difference. At any rate, with all the pharmaceutical, vitamin, and herbal aids out there, not to mention psychotherapy and counseling, no one should continue to suffer the debilitating effects of depression.

People with clinical depression should seek professional help immediately. If you've been feeling blue for more than a couple weeks, get help. (See Chapter 10 for more info.)

Here are some supplements that can help elevate your mood and even out your highs and lows:

✔ **Acetyl L-tyrosine:** Positive effects have been noted with acetyl L-tyrosine. Take 1,000–2,000 mg daily on an empty stomach. Take higher doses only under doctor supervision, because they can raise your blood pressure or lead to rapid pulse.

Do *not* take acetyl L-tyrosine with MAO inhibitor drugs, or if you tend to suffer from migraines. (Some MAO inhibitors include Bupropion, Harmaline, and Nardil.)

✔ **Black cohosh:** This helper reduces mood swings, anxiety, and depression, and hot flashes in postmenopausal women.

✔ **Damiana:** This medicinal plant is also supposed to be good for depression and anxiety. Take it three times a day as an *infusion* (herbal tea) or tincture.

✔ **Dandelion tea:** If you think suppressed anger is causing your depression, sip dandelion tea.

✔ **Folic acid:** People with a dietary deficiency of folic acid, part of the B vitamin complex, exhibit depressed mood, lethargy, poor concentration, and irritability. But studies suggest that taking folic acid supplements can help even if people aren't deficient. It seems to aid the response to antidepressant drugs, even in people who were previously unresponsive to medication. For some people, folic acid by itself may be enough to relieve depression. Take 500 mcg daily.

✔ **L-tryptophan:** Leading health experts highly recommend this amino acid. It helps the body increase its production of *serotonin,* the feel-good neurotransmitter that's often low in depressed people. Blood levels of tryptophan are also usually low in depressed people.

Take 2–4 grams of L-tryptophan daily. Take it before bedtime on an empty stomach. It works best if you also take niacinamide. Do *not* take tryptophan if you have asthma, because it can make your breathing problems worse.

✔ **NADH (nicotinamide adenine dinucleotide):** This *coenzyme* (active form of an enzyme system) plays a pivotal role in the body's energy production and can be safely combined with SAM-e. Start with 2.5 mg daily and increase your dosage by 2.5 mg each week until you find the right dose for you.

Don't take NADH too late in the day, because it can overstimulate you and prevent you from sleeping. Take it first thing in the morning on an empty stomach.

✔ **SAM-e (S-adenosyl-methionine):** Some evidence suggests that SAM-e (pronounced "Sammy") may be a fast-acting, safe, and effective antidepressant. It's an amino acid derivative that's normally synthesized in the body. It starts working in a week or two (sometimes in just a few days), compared to two to six weeks for prescription medication. Unlike medication, SAM-e doesn't come with a laundry list of side effects.

Start by taking one 200 mg tablet in the morning on an empty stomach. (Take it with food if it upsets your stomach; it won't work quite as effectively with food, so you may need to take a larger dose.) You can gradually increase the dosage up to 1,600 mg, depending on your needs. Generally, 400 mg seems to work. Be sure that the tablets are *enteric-coated;* if they aren't, your body won't absorb them properly. (Because the special coating can withstand stomach acid, enteric-coated tablets dissolve in the small intestine for maximum absorption.) Studies have shown that taking folic acid, B12, and B6 gives you even better protection against depression. Don't take SAM-e too late in the day, because it may interfere with your sleep.

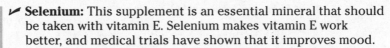

✔ **Selenium:** This supplement is an essential mineral that should be taken with vitamin E. Selenium makes vitamin E work better, and medical trials have shown that it improves mood.

✔ **St. John's Wort:** This supplement, which was widely used in Europe before gaining popularity in the United States, has received a lot of media play for its antidepressant effects. It's good for mild to moderate depression. You need to take it for four to six weeks or longer before starting to see any beneficial results. Make sure that you take capsules standardized to 0.3 percent hyperium. St. John's Wort may cause sun sensitivity.

✔ **Vitamin E:** This supplement can reduce mood swings. Make sure that you take the natural form, d-alpha (d'l-alpha is the synthetic form). The recommended dosage ranges from 400–1,600 IU daily. If you're diabetic or you have bleeding problems, you should talk to your physician before taking vitamin E in dosages more than 100 IU.

✔ **5-HTP:** This supplement may also be helpful in treating depression. Take 100 mg daily, or as recommended by your healthcare practitioner. See "Taking the Hypoglycemia Mix," earlier in this chapter for more information.

Digestive problems

You started eating the right foods, but your GI tract is throwing fits anyway. What can you do? Check out the following sections for some help.

Stomach

Eating the wrong foods, as well as eating them in far too large a quantity, causes many digestive problems. As you eat less of the foods that made you sick in the first place and turn to the recommended hypoglycemic diet (see Chapter 6), your digestive system will stop getting so overburdened.

Until this change in diet helps your condition improve, you can take licorice capsules before meals. (Don't confuse this supplement with licorice candy, which does you no good!) Taking two or three capsules about a half an hour before meals can prevent heartburn.

Digestive enzyme supplements can also help digestive problems. Choose enzyme capsules that include the following:

✔ **Amylase:** To help break down carbohydrates

✔ **Cellulose:** To digest fruits and vegetables

- **Lactase:** To digest milk
- **Lipase:** To break down fat
- **Protease:** To metabolize complex proteins

Eating a lot of cooked and processed foods can deplete your supply of natural digestive enzymes. This depletion may not matter so much when you're younger, but as you age and your supply of natural digestive enzymes diminishes, you'll find your system unable to properly digest foods or absorb nutrients. You're more apt then to suffer from the hallmarks of low blood sugar, such as decreased energy, headaches, and fatigue.

Liver

When considering digestion, you may have overlooked one organ: the liver. It's an underappreciated organ that slaves away each day, detoxifying your blood and ridding your body of poisonous substances. It's responsible for more than 500 functions. Secreting bile to aid in fat digestion is just one of these many functions.

When you have indigestion, your stomach isn't necessarily upset: It's often your liver. Well, you'd be upset, too, if no one ever thanked you for the all the work you do!

The least you can do is to give your liver some assistance. Here are some supplements to help:

- **Artichoke plant:** It isn't exactly an herb, but it's good for improving digestion and liver function. The part that's beneficial is the large basal leaf (everything but the heart). Clinical studies show that the basal leaves are good for digestion and liver function — what the studies neglect to mention is that they're also really delicious! Of course, it may be hard to eat an artichoke every day, even if you like them.

  A convenient way to enjoy the benefits of artichokes is to take an artichoke extract. (Black radish juice extract also encourages the liver to produce bile.) You can take 300–600 mg of standardized artichoke extract before, during, or after a meal. If you eat six small meals a day, though, you don't need to take the extract at each meal. Just take the extract whenever you need to, such as when you end up eating more than you want to. You should refrain from taking artichoke extract if you have gallstones or an obstruction of the bile duct.

- **Barberry:** Bitter compounds in barberry stimulate digestive function. It can also help fight infections and stomach problems.

- **Dandelion:** This herb aids digestion.

- ✔ **Elderflower:** This herb assists with digestion. It's also good for coughs, sore throats, fever, and hay fever.

- ✔ **Gentian:** This herb increases the numerous secretions along the entire digestive tract and helps get digestion back on track.

- ✔ **Milk thistle:** This herb has an active ingredient that's one of the strongest known liver protectors. It prevents toxins from damaging liver cells and speeds the healing of liver damage.

- ✔ **Peppermint:** Herbs in the mint family are excellent for digestion. Peppermint stimulates bile flow and the secretion of digestive juices.

- ✔ **Turmeric:** This bitter herb forms the base of most Indian curries. It's good for digestion, it helps build the blood, and it eases menstruation. It contains ingredients that are anti-inflammatory, antioxidant, and liver-protective.

Fatigue and energy drain

Everyone, especially people who have low blood sugar, experiences fatigue. A general feeling of fatigue isn't the same thing as Chronic Fatigue Syndrome (CFS). A diagnosis is critical but, generally speaking, you may have CFS if you have severe, unexplained fatigue that's not relieved by rest and that lasts for at least six or more consecutive months. (For more on CFS, see Chapter 3. For supplements that can help relieve the symptoms of CFS, see "Chronic fatigue syndrome," earlier in this chapter.)

For run-of-the-mill tiredness, you can try the following supplements:

- ✔ **Acetyl L-tyrosine:** This supplement is an amino acid. Take 1,000–2,000 mg daily.

  Don't take acetyl L-tyrosine if you're taking MAO inhibitor drugs or if you tend to suffer from migraines.

- ✔ **Lemon balm:** This herb calms, soothes, and revives energy.

- ✔ **Mint:** Herbs in the mint family can help revive energy.

- ✔ **Oatstraw:** This herb is a tonic that can relieve both physical and emotional fatigue. It's a good supplement to take when you're feeling frazzled and exhausted.

- ✔ **NADH (nicotinamide adenine dinucleotide):** This supplement is known as the "energizing coenzyme." It plays a crucial role in producing energy. With regular supplementation, you can expect to enjoy more energy and improved athletic performance. (See "Depression/mood swings," earlier in this chapter.)

- ✔ **Potassium:** This supplement is known to enhance energy and vitality. Take potassium aspartate with magnesium aspartate.

- ✔ **Siberian ginseng:** It can boost your energy but may be too strong if you have a weak constitution. You may have to take Siberian ginseng for several weeks before you feel an appreciable difference. When you take it, avoid caffeine and other stimulants.

- ✔ **Stinging nettle:** This herb is good for anemia, because it contains iron. It can also help with midafternoon slumps.

If you suffer from fatigue, be sure to rule out any possible medical causes. People with hypoglycemia sometimes have thyroid problems, so get your thyroid checked before trying the more potent herbs, such as Siberian ginseng.

Fibromyalgia

Fibromyalgia is estimated to afflict between 6 and 12 million people in the United States. It's a painful, debilitating syndrome that affects mostly women and bears a striking resemblance to chronic fatigue syndrome. Some people with hypoglycemia may also suffer from fibromyalgia. (Flip to Chapter 3 for more info.) For more on fibromyalgia, check out *Fibromyalgia For Dummies,* by Roland Staud, MD, and Christine Adamec (Wiley).

Intravenous vitamin and mineral injections may produce a significant improvement in the symptoms of fibromyalgia. For this type of treatment, consult a knowledgeable physician. The periodic use of UltraClear or UltraInflam detox programs, which are available through physicians, have also been known to help relieve the symptoms of fibromyalgia.

SAM-e, which is an anti-inflammatory that helps relieve muscular pain, and NADH (see "Depression/mood swings," earlier in this chapter) are also beneficial for treating the symptoms of fibromyalgia. If your condition is severe, you may want to try a gram dosage of SAM-e daily.

Headaches

Hypoglycemics often experience various types of headaches, ranging from mild to severe, in one or various parts of the head. Migraines are one kind of headache that can sometimes be triggered by a bout of low blood sugar. If you get headaches halfway between meals, they may be the result of having too much insulin in your bloodstream — which then leads to hypoglycemia.

You may be able to alleviate your headaches with the following remedies:

✔ **Feverfew:** This popular garden herb with its anti-inflammatory properties is beneficial for both arthritis and migraine headaches. Feverfew may help keep blood vessels from constricting, which can stop a throbbing headache.

Feverfew stimulates the uterus, so don't use it during pregnancy.

✔ **Fish oil capsules:** These are beneficial for the prevention of headaches. Unless you're allergic to fish, you should eat more cold-water fish, such as salmon, mackerel, and trout.

If you're pregnant, avoid fish unless otherwise instructed by your doctor.

✔ **Ginger:** Ginger prevents the release of substances that make blood vessels dilate. Keeping blood flow even can help prevent and relieve migraines. Use fresh or powdered ginger when you cook. You can also grate fresh ginger into juice.

✔ **Mullein:** This herb eases many kinds of lung ailments and strengthens the respiratory tract.

If correcting your blood sugar imbalance doesn't help relieve your headaches or if you have recurrent and/or severe headaches, get an appointment with your doctor.

Insomnia

Everyone needs some good, restful Zs. If you don't get them, you're bound to be listless, unfocused, and crabby. Inadequate or poor-quality sleep counts as *insomnia,* an underdiagnosed and under-treated sleep ailment. Insomnia can be a short-term (a single night to a few weeks), intermittent (episodes occur from time to time), or chronic (occurs most nights and lasts months or more) condition. If you suffer from insomnia, it may be caused by a serious illness, so don't wait to go to your friendly doctor.

If your insomnia isn't caused by an underlying illness, or if it's one of the symptoms of your hypoglycemia (and you should get a proper diagnosis for that, too), here are some things that can help:

✔ **Calcium:** Take it along with magnesium at night (in a ratio of 2 to 1). Take anywhere from 150–800 mg of calcium per day. Don't rely on milk alone, because it won't provide you with the correct amount of calcium.

✔ **Inositol:** A relative of the B-complex family, inositol has a calming effect and encourages sound sleep. For temporary insomnia, take 500–1,500 mg at bedtime. (Don't take any other B-complex vitamins at bedtime because they may keep you awake.)

✔ **Kava kava:** This herb is helpful for preventing insomnia.

Pregnant women should avoid kava kava, as should anyone with a liver condition.

✔ **Lettuce juice:** Some people find that drinking this juice helps them sleep better.

✔ **Niacin (B3):** This vitamin may be helpful if you fall asleep easily but can't go back to sleep after waking up in the middle of the night. Take 25–100 mg a day. You may experience a *niacin flush* (where you feel overheated and your face begins to redden) in the first few minutes after taking it. If you notice these flush symptoms, decrease your dosage or take *no-flush niacin,* which doesn't cause flushing.

✔ **Valerian:** Another herb that helps prevent insomnia. One study suggests that valerian root improved sleep for 80 percent of people with sleep problems.

Low sex drive

If you suffer from low blood sugar, you're also likely to experience low energy, which in turn leads to low sex drive. It's certainly not an uncommon symptom among hypoglycemics. Try the following:

✔ **Damiana:** This is reputed to amp up sexual interest for women when they sip it before bed. (But why restrict it to bedtime?) It's also supposed to alleviate depression and anxiety, two conditions that can dampen your sexual appetite. Take damiana three times a day as an infusion or a tincture.

✔ **Garlic:** Garlic breath may not exactly be an aphrodisiac, but eating garlic stimulates the hormone glands, which, in turn, revs up your sexual powers. Are you interested in finding out more? Garlic stimulates the central nerve of the penis and helps cause an erection. Garlic also nourishes and strengthens your entire body, giving you the stamina to romp a little longer in the hay.

The health-conscious Chinese use a lot of garlic in their cooking. (Come to think of it, maybe that's why they have a problem with overpopulation!) The Koreans eat a lot of garlic, too, and a low birth rate isn't one of their problems. Try garlic in your cooking and take garlic capsules so that you can maintain a consistent intake.

✔ **Nettle:** A highly concentrated extract from the nettle root is known to increase levels of free testosterone, which stimulates sex cell receptor sites in the brain.

✔ **Red clover:** The extract of this plant contains phytoestrogens, which can help maintain adequate estrogen levels in menopausal women, which in turn may improve the libido.

The Chinese regard the kidneys as the fountain of energy, and the kidneys and adrenal glands as the seat of sexuality. Anything that balances and strengthens the kidneys is good. Take daily doses of the following as tinctures to help your kidneys and adrenal glands:

✔ **Angelica:** This herb is also known as *dong quai* or *dang quai,* and is used in the East as a good female tonic. It's believed to help improve women's libido.

✔ **Chasteberry:** There's nothing chaste about this herb. It normalizes activity of the female sex hormones, and is especially beneficial during menopause.

✔ **Ginseng:** Ginseng has been used to boost energy and alertness in Asia for thousands of years. It contains compounds that invigorate sex drive and improve sex response and sex energy.

✔ **Saw palmetto:** It's been shown to be as effective in reducing a man's prostate gland as the prescription medication Proscar.

Memory problems/poor concentration

Problems with cognitive function are one of the key symptoms of hypoglycemia because the brain's only source of fuel is glucose. And when glucose levels are low — as in hypoglycemia — the brain doesn't work well. Without the necessary fuel, you're bound to have problems remembering anything or concentrating.

The following supplements can help improve your memory and concentration:

✔ **Choline:** The brain needs this substance to produce a major neurotransmitter.

✔ **Gingko tablets:** Gingko leaf extracts contain antioxidant properties. They also improve memory and alertness, and show promise in treating Alzheimer's disease.

✔ **Gotu kola:** Evidence indicates that gotu kola energizes the brain and improves concentration. Herbalists sometimes call this plant a vitamin for the brain.

✔ **Pantothenic acid:** Like choline, the brain needs it to facilitate the transmission of impulses between neurons.

✔ **Rosemary tea:** It's a handy-dandy way to perk you up anytime you're feeling dragged out. Drinking this tea is also a good way to start out the morning. Come to think of it, it's a good way to end the day, too.

Midafternoon slump

Grabbing some coffee and a sweet roll to help get out of the afternoon doldrums is all too easy. The caffeine and sugar duo — a double whammy — may perk you up, and you may even think that you're more productive, but don't kid yourself; you're only setting yourself up for a blood sugar crash to rival Black Monday's stock market crash. You'll be blue, and you'll be sorry, as you pay dearly for the teensy bit of indulgence. It's not worth it, especially when you have so many healthy alternatives.

For instance, you may want to try

✔ **Dandelion root tea:** This herb balances blood sugar and helps support liver function.

✔ **Ginseng:** This root is a good adrenal tonic that boosts energy. It's especially popular for increasing vitality and sexual energy. It also improves functioning of the lungs and stomach.

✔ **Gotu kola:** This herb accelerates the healing process, boosts memory, eases anxiety, increases energy, and protects against stress.

✔ **Grapefruit oil:** This supplement acts as a brisk refresher. It boosts memory and increases energy and mental ability. You can get it in teas, tinctures, and capsules.

✔ **Reishi:** This red mushroom strengthens the immune system and calms the nervous system. It can also help regulate blood sugar. Doctors often prescribe it for general weakness and fatigue.

✔ **Stinging nettle:** This popular mineral tonic is rich in vitamins and minerals. It can help heal inflamed mucous membranes caused by colds and coughs.

✔ **Yerba mate:** This South American herb is a great antioxidant that elevates mood and alertness without giving you the jitters. (But some people may object to the strong taste.)

Nausea

Ginger works well for nausea, motion sickness, morning sickness, and dizziness. It quells an upset stomach, reduces cholesterol, and strengthens the heart's overall functioning. For related conditions, see "Digestive problems," earlier in this chapter.

Poor circulation

Are you an ice princess or prince because of poor circulation? Remember to exercise regularly, because exercise (more than anything else) helps improve your circulation. Chapter 8 can get you moving in the right direction. In addition, you may also want to try the following:

- ✔ **Cinnamon and cayenne pepper:** Sprinkle ground cinnamon and cayenne pepper into your socks and gloves (they should preferably be made of cotton) to increase circulation and help warm cold hands and feet.

  Be careful not to get cayenne in your eyes! Wash your hands thoroughly before touching yourself — or anyone else. If your skin is sensitive, don't touch the pepper with bare hands.

- ✔ **Garlic:** Eat more garlic. (So what doesn't garlic do?) If you can't eat garlic for any reason, then take it in the form of garlic pills, but get it into your system somehow.

- ✔ **Ginger:** Add ginger to your cooking, or grind it up and steep it as tea. Ground ginger in bottles is okay for cooking and flavoring, but it's generally not potent enough for healing purposes.

- ✔ **Warming foods:** Eating warming foods, such as healthy soups, may help your circulation. Drink your beverages at room temperature or warmer. (Try to avoid iced beverages.) Refrain from eating raw vegetables until your body becomes *hotter* — when it's stronger and circulation has improved. (Not everyone agrees with this view. Raw foodists — people who consume mostly raw foods — believe that raw vegetables can help heat up people who appear to be constitutionally cold.)

  In traditional Chinese medicine, people with a weak constitution who tend to suffer from cold hands and feet are told to avoid eating raw vegetables because they have a cooling effect on the body. Instead of eating cold salads, try quickly steaming your salads — for only a minute or two, so as not to destroy the nutrients. Rather than eat fruits or yogurts straight from the fridge, leave them out for awhile so they're not ice-cold to the touch. (But don't leave them out so long that they become spoiled. Making sure that food doesn't spoil is especially important in the summer.)

Stress

When it comes to vitamins, supplements, and herbs, just about anything that improves your overall health or strengthens the functioning of any organ helps combat stress.

 An anti-stress vitamin regimen should include the B-complex vitamins, vitamin C, vitamin E, magnesium, calcium, potassium, chromium, manganese, selenium, and iron. Specifically, keep the following supplements in mind (and mouth):

- **Astral:** This herb is a good tonic. It supports the immune system and helps the adrenal glands deal with stress.

- **Ginseng:** This famous herb helps you adapt to just about any physiological stress. It helps restore equilibrium when your body has been thrown out of whack by stressors. Siberian ginseng enhances overall physical endurance. Korean ginseng is good, too, but its effects may be a little too potent.

- **Mugwort:** This herb, available in liquid or tea form, is often prescribed for stress. You can take it as a tincture or place ½ ounce of dried herb in half a cup of water.

 Use caution if you have hay fever or are allergic to hazelnuts. Avoid it if you're pregnant or on blood thinners.

- **Pantothenic acid:** This vitamin is required for the adrenal glands to work properly. If you're very stressed, take more than 700 mg daily in single or divided doses.

- **Pyridoxine (vitamin B6):** This vitamin helps with the synthesis of the neurochemicals important for counteracting stress. Take the same dosage of other B-complex vitamins.

 Don't take more than 100 mg, however, because excessive doses can cause nerve damage.

- **Reishi mushrooms:** These mushrooms are an excellent tonic. They give you a sense of overall well-being.

 Refrain from taking too many of these mushrooms, especially if you're still young, because their effect is very strong. As with anything, you need to find a good balance.

You may also want to consider the relaxing herbs, such as the popular chamomile, lavender, valerian, lemon balm, passionflower, hops, and California poppy.

Water retention

You may experience water retention as a result of your hypoglycemia (or for a variety of other reasons).

If water retention is so severe that pressing on a swollen spot leaves indentations on your skin, go see your doctor immediately. Otherwise, you may want to try one of the following remedies to help relieve your discomfort:

- **Diuretic herbs:**
  - Corn silk tea is a safe and effective diuretic. But don't sip it at night, because it'll make you go to the bathroom.
  - Nettle and dandelion also have diuretic properties.
- **Water:** Drinking more water can help relieve water retention, especially if you also cut back on sodium.

Taking a Whiff: Aromatherapy

Because the *limbic system* (which includes the brain's hypothalamus, hippocampus, and amygdala; the limbic system is especially concerned with emotion and motivation) processes odor and emotions, smells evoke powerful and immediate reactions. *Aromatherapy,* using essential oils for therapeutic purposes, is a good addition in soothing hypoglycemia's physical and emotional effects, and smoothing your transition to a healthier lifestyle.

Essential oils are the aromatic and volatile liquids derived from herbs or plants. Because essential oils are highly aromatic, you can get many of their benefits by simply inhaling or diffusing them into the room. Buy only pure, natural essential oils if you want the full range of physical and psychological benefits of aromatherapy.

After you get used to handling the oils, they're quite safe. But as with anything, including prescription medicine, treat them with precaution. Be aware of the following essential oil don'ts:

- Don't take essential oils by mouth, because they can be quite toxic. If you accidentally swallow an essential oil, call your local poison control center (keep the number in a handy place) or 911 immediately.
- Don't get the oil in your eyes or on other sensitive body parts.

✔ Don't let children or pets near essential oils.

✔ Don't ever apply any of the essential oils directly to your skin without first diluting them. The oils are very concentrated, and they will irritate your skin.

✔ Don't forget to consult a knowledgeable healthcare practitioner before using any essential oils. If you suffer from serious or chronic illnesses, such as cancer, epilepsy, heart disease, or asthma, be very careful about using essential oils; their potency is nothing to sniff at.

If you have very sensitive skin or allergies, do a patch test before using an essential oil. Dab a 2-percent solution of the essential oil and water on a small patch of skin, such as the underside of your arm. Over the next 12 hours, check for any redness or itching. If you notice either, don't use the oil on your skin. Even if you can't apply the diluted oil to your skin, you can still dab it on a tissue, hankie, or cotton ball and inhale it as needed. You can also put a few drops in your bath.

If you really want to get into aromatherapy heavy duty, several books on the subject are available, including *Aromatherapy For Dummies,* by Kathi Keville (Wiley). You can also find out more from a reputable aromatherapist. Ask for referrals for trained, certified aromatherapists from people you trust.

Rocking Bach's Flower Remedies

This is true flower power! The theory behind flower remedies is that the energy of flowers contained in *flower essences* (the extract from flowers) treats emotional patterns that result in the manifestation of physical symptoms. One of the most popular formulas, Bach's Rescue Remedy, is reputed to be quite effective for stress. Some people even use flower essences for their pets.

Right now, virtually no scientific studies back up the claims of flower-essence healing, mostly because the essences don't lend themselves readily to scientific research. So, although they're fun to try, be careful and controlled in your experiments, and know that essential oils and flower essences can't replace advice from a doctor. When in doubt, always consult a healthcare practitioner.

Part III
Emulating Lifestyles of the Well and Healthy

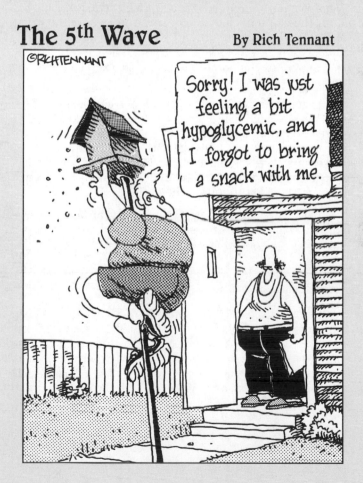

In this part . . .

*I*n this part, we help you map out a lifestyle for achieving the vibrant health you desire. You explore the wonderful world of movement, and you figure out how to
choose exercises that are fun for you. When you're ready
to rev your body up, there's nothing like exercise. Now it's
time to get rolling.

This part shows you how trendy hypoglycemia really is.
It's what you might call a lifestyle disease — a condition
aggravated by an unhealthy style of living. You discover
how to manage stress and deal with the old demon,
depression. Stress is especially relevant to hypoglycemia,
because many of the signs and symptoms of hypoglycemia
are caused by disruptions in the stress hormones.

This part also provides helpful tips to get through a stressful (and even a not-so-stressful) day at work — the place
where you spend a lot of your time.

Chapter 8

Easing Symptoms and Energizing with Exercise

*E*nergy is probably the last thing you feel when your body and brain cells aren't properly fueled, right? What's more, as a hypoglycemic, you've probably been chronically undernourished, so the weakness lingers. You must balance your blood sugar to properly fuel your body.

However, before you run out, buy a new exercise wardrobe, and sign up for a lifetime gym membership, take a deep breath. You need to start small and gradually incorporate exercise into your lifestyle. This chapter can help you relieve some of your hypoglycemia symptoms with aerobic activities, yoga and T'ai Chi, weightlifting, and other forms of exercise. You can make your life a little more manageable. Before you start exercising, first read this chapter.

Why Exercise Is Important When Battling Hypoglycemia

Unfortunately, you can't balance your blood sugar and properly fuel your body by using a quick fix; permanent lifestyle changes are the only way to go. Changing your diet is the first step. Chapter 6 helps you do that. The next step is getting regular exercise. Exercise goes hand in hand with diet changes, and it's crucial for improved health and well-being. Exercise helps you

  ✔ **Battle depression.** Depression is a major hypoglycemia symptom that *endorphins,* which are released when you're active, can work to fight. Endorphins are feel-good hormones produced by the body. They're nature's own painkillers.

✔ **Gain insulin sensitivity.** Increased sensitivity results in lower blood insulin levels. (Chapter 2 gives you details about how hypoglycemia works.)

✔ **Boost self-confidence.** This boost includes better body image and more control over other aspects of life.

✔ **Achieve and maintain your ideal weight.** This is another critical issue for a hypoglycemic. (Chapter 6 has more info.)

✔ **Stick to a healthy diet.** After you get into shape, your body will desire good carbs, protein, fruits, and vegetables.

✔ **Become stronger and healthier.** When you're strong and healthy, you don't need to be quite as compulsive about your diet. You can eat more carbs, and you can even eat forbidden foods on occasion without suffering undue consequences.

Understanding why exercise is important doesn't mean you can go out tomorrow morning and run three miles. Before you start any exercise program, keep the following points in mind:

✔ **Always see a doctor before participating in a fitness program.** (Chapter 4 gives you doc-picking info.)

✔ **Pick an activity that you're suited for and that appeals to you.** No matter what the activity is, pick something that you enjoy doing because it can keep you more motivated. If you pick something that you dread, chances are you won't stick with it when you get bored.

✔ **Enjoy many activities.** Do a variety of exercises to keep from getting bored. As a matter of fact, a variety is good because you work different parts of your body.

✔ **If you already have an exercise routine but you're not getting the results you want, review it.** Keeping track of your progress in your food journal (Chapter 6) is a good way to start. Write down the activity along with the intensity and duration.

If you never vary your routine, your body adapts, and you stop making progress. To avoid this plateau, make small, continual changes.

If you're completely out of shape or haven't exercised for years, don't suddenly start a vigorous program of exercise. You're likely to hurt yourself. Check with your doctor before you start any program. If you want more general knowledge and comprehensive guidance on how to get fit, check out *Fitness For Dummies,* 3rd Edition, by Susanne Schlosberg and Liz Neporent (Wiley).

Easing Your Way into Exercise

What if you can't stomach the thought of exercise? Even if exercise doesn't excite you, gradually adding just a bit of exercise to your daily routine can help relieve your hypoglycemia symptoms and help you feel better.

No matter what exercise you decide to do, one possible solution is to combine it with something you enjoy. For instance, if you like to zone out in front of the tube, why not exercise while you're watching TV? It may keep you more alert and better conditioned than you've ever been. To ease into exercise, you can begin by walking in place, and then gradually add running in place. Just imagine, you'll be getting a good workout while enjoying your favorite show! Needless to say, you don't have to stick to TV — you can just as easily do your workouts while listening to books, lectures, or seminars on CDs or media content players.

Not sure how to start? This section helps you make that transition to exercise by first modifying your behavior and then finding the time to exercise regularly. In no time at all, you can begin to feel better.

Modifying your behavior

One way to gradually condition yourself to exercise is through a behavior modification technique that psychologists call *approximation*. For example, if your objective is to exercise by walking on the treadmill, then start by simply getting on the treadmill and standing on it for five minutes every day. To make the activity more appealing, try reading the paper or a magazine, or sipping an unsweetened beverage while standing on the treadmill. After that, walk for two minutes. Gradually increase the time on the treadmill every week until you're walking for at least 20 minutes.

When walking in place, bringing your knees up higher increases the aerobic intensity. To vary the routine, you can jump from side to side, add a few jumping jacks, or skip with an imaginary rope. You can also alternate walking with jumping or running in place. Working up quite a sweat is possible just by doing these simple exercises — without ever losing sight of your TV! After you get used to this special "couch potato" exercise routine, your body will become better toned. At that time you may discover that you're ready — perhaps even eager — to go outside for a walk or a jog, or join an exercise class or two. An interesting phenomenon about fitness is that when you become more physically fit, you actually start craving exercise.

Finding the time to exercise

You work 40-plus hours a week. You have two kids (or grandkids) to run to volleyball practice and piano lessons. You have household chores to do. Are you wondering how anyone can fit in exercise?

The optimum amount of exercise for people suffering from chronic ailments, such as hypoglycemia, is an hour a day, for a minimum of five days a week. That may sound daunting, but even ultra-fast workouts of five to ten minutes a day, a couple times a day, can be a great start. These speed workouts can be highly effective. If you haven't exercised much in the past, these exercises will undoubtedly invigorate you.

If you're already in shape, you can most likely jump to the next level of fitness by either adding the ultra-fast exercises to your basic workout routine or incorporating them as modifications to the basic regimen. Focused, intensive training for brief amounts of time can be more effective than an hour or more of halfheartedly dragging out a workout. And doing something — anything — for even five to ten minutes a day is better than doing nothing. But the truth is that if you want to obtain optimum health and fitness, five to ten minutes a day isn't enough.

After you incorporate short bursts of exercise into your day, look for ways to add longer periods of exercise into your daily routine. If you're busy, you probably don't have large chunks of idle time.

The easy solution is to break up your workout sessions. Do ten-to-fifteen-minute workouts several times a day. For instance, exercise for ten minutes when you first get up to rev you up and get you going. Work out once more in the mid-morning or before lunch, and then again immediately after work (this helps you unwind after a long day), and so forth. (You can do light stretching late at night but refrain from vigorous exercise because that can hinder sleep.) Studies have shown that you can get the same benefits and similar conditioning with these shorter bursts of exercise as long as they add up to at least half an hour (ideally an hour) a day.

Timing Your Carbs

The subject of carbohydrates is of vital importance to anyone who's struggling with erratic blood sugar levels. That's because carbs most directly affect the sugar in your blood. (For a complete discussion on carbs and blood sugar, see Chapters 2 and 6.) The short version? When you begin exercising, hormones are released into the bloodstream signaling the liver and fat cells to liberate their stored energy nutrients, primarily glucose. How much *glycogen* (the sugar your body stores) you have in store depends partly on the amount of carbs in your diet. When you exercise, your body uses up a lot of glucose, which needs replenishing. You need to know what to eat and when to eat it to prevent a blood sugar crash.

Studies have shown that eating carbs an hour before exercising can extend endurance and improve performance. If you're going to take part in a strenuous form of exercise for more than 90 minutes, such as mountain climbing, cross-country skiing, aerobics, or gym workouts, your best bet is to eat a meal containing carbs about one to two hours before the event. Doing so allows time for the food to leave the stomach and reach the small intestine. You don't want to eat too close to your workout; otherwise, food will still be in your stomach, and you may get nauseated.

On the other hand, if you eat about two hours or more before your workout, most of the carbs will have already been burned up. The trick, therefore, is to eat something that's very slowly digested and absorbed so that it remains in the intestine hours after consumption.

Which carbs should you choose? Select foods with a GI (glycemic index) of less than 55. (Check out www.glycemicindex.com for more info on food with a low GI.) The body needs carbs as fuel, but eating foods with a lower GI will spare you problems. After an intense workout, however, a high GI food can help to restore the glycogen in muscles in time for the next event. If you're not a particularly athletic person, and you don't regularly participate in events, you don't need to worry so much about replenishing your glycogen store. If you're famished after exercise, eat something that quickly restores your blood sugar, and follow that with a lower-GI carbohydrate and a little bit of protein.

Improving Insulin and Feeling the Burn: Aerobics

Aerobic literally means *with air*. Aerobic activity increases your body's air intake, allowing you to burn more calories. Aerobic exercise is any activity that gets your heart pumping faster and your lungs taking in more oxygen. Walking, bicycling, swimming, stair climbing — and yes, sex — count as aerobic exercise. But don't rely exclusively on sex as a fitness regimen.

Fun in the sun

Did you know that a growing body of research suggests that exposure to natural light for one and a half to two hours a day may activate the adrenal glands and thereby support adrenal function? Because the adrenals are involved with normal blood sugar regulation, people with low blood sugar may do well to get some sun every day.

A really good way to get some sunlight is to exercise outdoors. Not only is it invigorating, but it also helps your body acclimatize to the changing seasons better. Better overall health can also translate into better blood sugar regulation. But you need to watch out for bad air days and remember the following tips to stay safe:

✔ If there's a pollution alert, don't needlessly expose yourself.

✔ Don't jog in the smog.

✔ Apply sunscreen that blocks both UVA and UVB rays and has an SPF rating of at least 15.

✔ Don't wear perfume in the sun, because some perfumes contain ingredients that can cause burns or rashes when exposed to sunlight. Besides, the mix of perfume and sweat isn't the most alluring scent.

✔ Wear a helmet if you're participating in an activity that requires one (such as biking), especially if you're prone to dizzy spells from attacks of low blood sugar.

Most fitness experts agree that the best workout combines aerobic activity with some form of weight training. (For more info on weightlifting, check out "Kicking Weakness with Weights" later in this chapter.) For most people, the optimal amount of exercise is one hour per day, five to seven days per week. Exercising for longer than a one-hour period may be counterproductive because your body may begin to produce *cortisol,* a stress hormone. In addition, exercising for too long, especially without fueling up, may itself result in a bout of low blood sugar.

So do you want to start the burning? This section is a good place to begin. You can read more about walking, running, jogging, and even dancing.

Strut your stuff and work that walk

Walking is a simple and easy activity that just about anybody can do, which makes it one of the best exercises for improving your health. Walking makes the body more sensitive to the effects of insulin and thus allows more glucose to be absorbed by the cells.

Any exercise that improves insulin function is good for people who have problems metabolizing glucose or regulating blood sugar.

Walking has been proven to help people reduce their cravings for addictive substances, such as nicotine, alcohol, and barbiturates. If you're hypoglycemic, one of the worst things you can do is abuse a substance like liquor or tobacco, but when you're addicted, quitting is hard to do. Use walking as your tool for fighting those cravings and keeping your hypoglycemia under control.

Walking, an aerobic workout, is especially good for the blood-sugar challenged, because walking is easy to start and maintain (even if you're suffering from fatigue), and it doesn't have complex routines to memorize (if you're suffering from brain fog). If you're out of shape, or if you've been otherwise inactive for a long time, walking may be the best way for you to begin exercising. After you exercise with walking for a while, you can simply continue with it, complement it with other activities, or use it as a transitional activity for other sports.

Here are some walking do's:

- **Before a walk that will last an hour or more, do eat a snack with some protein and a complex carb.** For example, eat a half a slice of whole grain bread with nut butter or raw (or lightly steamed) broccoli dipped in miso paste. These snacks ensure that your blood sugar doesn't drop mid-track.

- **Do carry a snack and a water bottle with you.** Hypoglycemics should always carry food in the event that your blood sugar dips too low. You should also avoid getting dehydrated.

- **Do use exercise walking, which combines arm and leg movements.** *Fitness Walking For Dummies,* by Liz Neporent (Wiley), informs you of every aspect of walking.

- **Do get the right shoes.** Your shoes should be flexible, have breathable fabrics, and provide good traction. Look for cushioning at the tongue, around the collar, and at the heel. If you walk fast, look for cushioning at the ball of the foot, also.

- **If you tend to get dizzy or tire easily, do walk at night rather than in the morning.** In the morning your blood sugar is lower.

- **Do get a weighted vest.** They're specially designed for walking, and you can get one that allows you to increase the weight as you become better conditioned. The weights increase resistance and help you burn more calories. Most people can start out with low weights in the vest, but if you're very much out of shape, don't wear a vest until you're in better shape.

Now that you know what to do, check out these walking don'ts to make sure you stay safe:

✔ **Don't walk while wearing ankle or wrist weights.** You may injure yourself from the added strain. (Weighted vests apply the weight more evenly and are therefore less likely to cause problems.)

✔ **Don't wear weights (vest or otherwise) that are more than 10 percent of your body weight.** You may otherwise develop back problems.

✔ **Don't forget to replace your walking shoes every 400 miles (or when they start showing wear).** Worn-out shoes don't provide enough support to protect your knees or lower back.

What's the difference, you ask? Running and jogging

Running and jogging (a slower version of running) are good exercises, and they're darn good ways to get your blood circulating and burn up calories. However, if you have low blood pressure — as many hypoglycemics do — and if bouts of low blood sugar have left you wearier than not, it may be too much to suddenly start running. A good workout combination is running and walking. For instance, walk fast for 10 minutes, run for 1 minute, and then walk at a normal pace for another 10 minutes.

For maximum aerobic benefit, jog for at least 20 minutes at your *target heart rate*. The target rate shows you how fast your heart should beat per minute when you exercise. To calculate your individual heart rate:

1. **Subtract your age from 226 if you're a woman, and 220 if you're a man.**

   For example, say that you're a 96-year-old man. Take 220–96 to get 124.

2. **Multiply the result by .70.**

   This is your maximum target heart rate. In the example, take the 124×.70 to get 86.8, your maximum target heart rate.

3. **Multiply the result by .80.**

   This is your minimum target heart rate. To finish the example, take your maximum heart rate (86.8) and multiply it by .80 to get 69.44, your minimum target heart rate.

Don't worry if you can't maintain your target heart rate for 20 minutes. Recent studies have shown that you can get similar benefits with even 5-minute workouts interspersed at various times of the day. And if you can't get outside to run, run in place; the intensity won't be the same, but anything is better than sitting on your butt.

As with most exercises that involve your feet, shoes are an extremely important part of running. The proper shoes ensure that you get the most out of your workout and avoid injury. You can read more about what to look for in shoes in this chapter's previous section, and you can also buy your running shoes from a store that specializes in runners' needs. With this type of store, you can use the knowledge of the experts to be sure that you're buying the best shoes for your feet.

Shaking your groove thang: Dancing

You don't need to boogie all night to get the benefits of dance. This fantastic activity can make you chipper, dapper, and slimmer — *and* it can lift you right up from the doldrums of the low blood sugar blues. And you're not limited to any one kind of dance. You can choose from all different types of dance: jazz, modern, hip-hop, African, belly, and folk, to name just a few. You can do it solo, in a pair, or as a group. (For a specific example of how to incorporate dance into your life, check out the nearby sidebar, "Bust a move with a dance program.")

Bust a move with a dance program

If you're tired of dancing to the same old beat, or if you're just looking for something different, consider trying a dance program, such as the Neuromuscular Integrative Action (NIA) dance program.

NIA is adaptable to every age and body type, and for all levels of physical fitness. Practitioners describe NIA as "fusion fitness" because NIA combines nonimpact aerobics, dance, yoga-like movement, and some elements of martial arts. NIA lends itself easily to solo or group dancing.

NIA's adherents believe that regular participation can help improve blood circulation, strengthen the immune system, and even alleviate emotional problems and anxiety disorders. Of course, many other exercise and activity programs may provide similar benefits. What's important is that you choose an activity that you enjoy doing and that's right for your fitness level.

Find out more by visiting NIA's Web site at http://nia-nia.com. You can find NIA classes worldwide through this site.

Whether you're married or single, you can add a little oomph into your love life by dancing as a couple or getting your body revved up with dance. But what does this oomph have to do with low blood sugar? Plenty! When you're so often weary, down in the dumps, or crabby as a result of your hypoglycemia, love and lust can leach away and fizzle down to a most unfortunate finale. So if your hypoglycemic syndrome has put a strain in your relationship, what better way to put the sparkle back than through dance? (Chapters 13 and 14 address relationship issues at length.)

If you've been sidelined by hypoglycemia for a long time, don't overdo it; ease yourself into any new activity. Find a class that's appropriate to your fitness level. Ballroom dancing and folk dance are generally pretty safe choices. Make sure that you tell your instructor about any physical or medical problems you may have.

Regulating Blood Sugar with Yoga and T'ai Chi

Yoga and T'ai Chi (and related forms) are specifically designed to promote mental, emotional, and spiritual growth along with physical fitness. Although quite different in practice, T'ai Chi and yoga do have similarities. They're both comprehensive forms of exercise that work the entire body, tone and build muscles, strengthen the organs and musculoskeletal structure, and improve circulation of the *qi* (also spelled ch'i) — the life force that courses through the body.

Both T'ai Chi and yoga fit well into *comprehensive treatment* programs for diabetes and hypoglycemia that involve mind, body, and spirit. These ailments have a genetic component, but other contributing factors are diet, sedentary habits, and physical, emotional, and mental stress. All these factors are addressed in a holistic manner in the practices of T'ai Chi and yoga. (Chapter 4 talks more about holistic and Eastern approaches, as well.)

So which should you study? It depends on what you like, what feels most comfortable to you, and the instructors you can find. This section can help you.

Going yoga

Yoga, which started in India, consists of poses you hold from a few seconds to several minutes. Many forms, such as Hatha yoga and

Iyengar yoga, exist. Most forms include the same fundamental poses, but some classes focus more on sweating, some on breathing, and some on spirituality.

Numerous studies have reported the beneficial effect of yoga on regulating blood sugar control. Some even venture to claim that some cases of type 1 diabetes (what used to be known as *juvenile diabetes*) were controlled through yoga. (Chapter 3 has more info on diabetes.) The direct stimulation of the pancreas by certain yogic postures seems to stimulate and rejuvenate the pancreatic cells, which are responsible for producing insulin. Although the studies only dealt with the effect on diabetes, the findings suggest by implication that yoga is beneficial for hypoglycemia.

If you're interested in trying yoga, check out *Yoga For Dummies,* by Georg Feuerstein, Larry Payne, and Lilias Folan for a good starter, or *Yoga with Weights For Dummies,* by Sherri Baptiste and Megan Scott (both by Wiley) if you want to discover how to safely combine working out with free weights while practicing yoga poses.

Taking T'ai Chi

T'ai Chi Chuan (also spelled "Taiji") has often been described as Chinese yoga. Because T'ai Chi is a set of smooth, flowing exercises, people tend to forget that it's a martial art. Although T'ai Chi actively discourages violence, you can learn fighting skills, such as sparring and self-defense. T'ai Chi is a *soft,* or internal, form of martial arts (as opposed to the *hard* external schools, such as Shaolin, karate, or Tae Kwon Do). Unlike the hard schools of martial arts, T'ai Chi is accessible to elderly or frail people, but it can also be rigorous and demanding.

Unless you already have a background in martial arts, don't attempt to learn T'ai Chi from a video. Unlike aerobics or dance, learning T'ai Chi properly without the physical presence of a qualified instructor is extremely difficult, if not impossible. If you try to learn T'ai Chi without an instructor, you'll likely pick up bad habits that will be hard to correct later on. Do yourself a favor and find a class and instructor who you really like.

The best way to find a class you like is to get recommendations from people you trust. You can also visit the Guang Ping Yang Tai chi Chuan Web site (www.guangpingyang.org) and find a listing of certified instructors. For more specific suggestions, check out *T'ai Chi For Dummies,* by Therese Iknoian (Wiley). For a good beginning introduction to T'ai Chi, go to www2.gol.com/users/ddh where you can read free articles.

Although hydration is important when exercising, don't drink liquids for at least 15 minutes before practicing T'ai Chi. Avoid eating 30 minutes before and after practice. Unless you're extremely dehydrated, avoid drinking water (especially if the water's cold) during the practice. Drinking liquids can cool your body and damper the really good flow of qi that your workout sets in motion.

Kicking Weakness with Weights

Exercising with weights may be very effective and helpful for people who have problems with blood sugar balance. Good muscle tone seems to improve cell ability to make good use of insulin and to help the body regulate blood sugar levels.

You don't need to become a muscle-bound lifter to benefit from weight training. Building and toning muscle is one of the most effective ways to boost your metabolism, lose weight, and increase bone density (which can help stave off osteoporosis) for hypoglycemics and non-hypoglycemics alike.

Despite the claims of some high-profile exercise gurus, bodyweight exercises don't necessarily yield the same or better results compared to lifting free weights or using weight machines. Different exercises and techniques will yield different results for different people. One exercise, or one way of doing it, isn't necessarily better or worse than another.

If you're interested in working with weights, this section can get you started by first explaining how bodyweight workouts can help and then by explaining how you can ease into using free weights. For more info, you can also check out *Weight Training For Dummies,* 3rd Edition, by Liz Neporent, Suzanne Schlosberg, and Shirley J. Archer (Wiley).

Building endurance with bodyweight workouts

Bodyweight exercises use your full body weight, or as much of it as possible, for resistance. They build and tone muscles to increase your stamina, and to improve your overall conditioning. You can do bodyweight exercises anytime, anywhere, with no special equipment or facilities. Although bodyweight exercises aren't new, they're enjoying a recent surge of interest among people who want the benefit of weight-bearing or weight-resistance exercises without the hassle of buying and using free weights or going to the gym.

If you're suffering from chronic hypoglycemia, bodyweight exercises are a good way to start building muscle mass and tone to help body cells use insulin more effectively. This kind of exercise will help keep your hypoglycemia from progressing to the next stage, insulin resistance. (Flip to Chapter 3 for more.)

Bodyweight exercises are easier to get started with than traditional weight-lifting regimens. In addition, they require no additional equipment, and individuals may feel less resistance (no pun intended) about doing these exercises.

Some examples of bodyweight exercises include

- Push-ups
- Pull-ups
- Squats
- Calisthenics
- Gymnastic movements, such as the *planche* (a movement involving arching of the body) and the *front lever* (a movement involving hollowing of the body)
- Yoga

If you've never worked out before, start with easy, basic exercises such as push-ups or leg raises. Any one of the preceding exercises is suitable. If you know nothing about exercise, enroll in a good class so that you can discover how to do the movements properly, without injuring yourself.

Advocates of bodyweight exercises typically emphasize the importance of repetition. For example, doing 100 or even 500 squats definitely teaches you something about endurance! As with any exercise, the key is to start slow and gradually build up to the desired number of repetitions. (*Note:* Some trainers advise against doing more than 150 repetitions of any exercise on a regular basis. Moderation helps avoid the possibility of causing a repetitive stress or strain injury.)

Calisthenics typically involve movement against relatively little weight resistance. Examples include swinging your arms in circles or touching your toes. Calisthenics work against much less of your body weight than typical bodyweight exercises.

Many people effectively combine calisthenics, gymnastic movements, and even yoga with other exercises in their workout routines. There's little point in arguing about what is or isn't bodyweight exercise — if you have time to be arguing, you're better off exercising!

Easing into free weights with body weights

When you're feeling fitter and can bid adieu to hypoglycemic symptoms, you can transition into actually working with free weights or weight machines if you want to.

 Before you start actually using free weights or weight machines, make sure you get guidance from a professional. You can find a lot of information and misinformation out there. For example, fitness and weight-lifting magazine articles are frequently intended more to sell products rather than to inform. In some cases, the buffed-up models gracing the magazine pages may not have even tried the product or program they're selling. Don't be fooled by the glossy sales and marketing techniques.

 Make sure you have a *spotter* (someone to help you lift the dumb-bell on and off the rack) when you're working with weights. Spotters can help you if you have trouble completing a set and keep you from getting hurt. And don't be too cavalier when handling dumbbells and other weights.

In addition to helping spot you, a personal trainer or qualified person from your gym can ensure that you're getting the proper workout and that you're correctly using the weights. Make sure that you know how to lift weights correctly before lifting them solo at home, unless you're using only 1- to 5-pound dumbbells. Even then, proper training is important.

Don't be misled by high-profile exercise gurus or self-styled "fitness celebrities" flogging expensive DVDs, CDs, books, Web sites with hefty membership fees, and so on. The same information may be available elsewhere for free (for example, try a simple Internet search or visit your local public library). You don't have to spend big bucks to get into shape. Balancing and regulating your blood sugar and keeping yourself healthy are more about sticking to your diet and regular exercise program.

Incorporating free weights into your exercise regimen

 Make sure that you consult your doctor before you begin any exercise regimen. This caveat is true for anyone, but particularly for individuals who suffer from chronic health conditions like hypoglycemia. You can hurt yourself if you get dizzy during a workout session.

Proceed slowly when incorporating free weights. Start with dumb-bells weighing about 1.5 to 3 pounds, depending on your gender and fitness level. (Men can generally lift more weight than women.) Using lighter weights is safer and can be just as effective as heavier weights if you do enough repetitions. You can combine a few free weight exercises (such as bicep curls) with your aerobic or other exercise regimen. For example, you may do some resistance exercises before or after an aerobic workout. In the beginning, don't lift weights for longer than 10 or 15 minutes.

You can gradually increase the time, as well as the weights. Because each person is so different, we can't map out an exercise plan that will suit everyone. For best results, keep an exercise log and vary your routine so you cover all parts of the body.

Clearing Brain Fog with Qigong

Brain fog is mental confusion, a feeling that often accompanies hypoglycemia. (For more on brain fog, see Chapter 3.) And what is *qigong?* Simply put, it's a Chinese system of physical training, phi-losophy, and comprehensive preventive and therapeutic health-care that involves breathing exercises and meditation. It's somewhat related to T'ai Chi and other soft forms of martial arts, but it doesn't have any of the hard elements of martial arts, such as kicks and strikes. (For more info on the various forms of martial arts, see the nearby sidebar, "Mastering the martials.")

The *qi* in qigong refers to breath, vital essence, and life force; *gong* means skill, work, and self-discipline. Many scientific studies have been done on the numerous benefits of qigong. Most importantly for hypoglycemics, qigong has been found to help regulate blood sugar by strengthening the *endocrine system,* blood sugar's regulator.

You can use qigong to gain, attain, and maintain vibrant health, helping to strengthen the body. Qigong can also strengthen the blood and immune system and energize the brain. If you do it right, you'll be better able to sense your body, which can help you tune in to the diet your body actually needs, rather than to what an out-side authority or some school of thought tells you.

There are more than 3,000 varieties of qigong. Proper instruction is important (just like T'ai Chi, you can't really learn qigong through a book or a video, although you can use those tools as supplements), and so is regular practice. You need to have patience, persistence, and commitment to enjoy the full benefits of qigong. Give qigong a minimum of three months and up to a year before expecting to see any changes. If you want to find out more information about qigong, check out the National Qigong Association site (www.nqa.org), purchase or rent qigong DVDs, or sit in on a qigong class.

Be aware that many charlatans claim to be qigong masters. We can't give you a formula for telling who's legitimate and who's not. Try to get personal recommendations. Generally, beware of anyone who claims to be able to heal everything under the sun with only a few exercises, especially if the person charges an exorbitant fee for his classes or services.

Avoid sexual intercourse for at least one hour before and after a qigong session. Having sex an hour before or after a session may interfere with your training because it can impede the flow of qi.

Mastering the martials

Studying the fighting arts for your health is something you may want to consider. Through the practice, you'll cultivate discipline, commitment, self-confidence, strength, and directness of purpose — the diametric opposite of how you are when weak and debilitated by your system's metabolic glitch. It'll definitely clear any cobwebs in your brain and make your thinking sharp. You'll hardly remember what brain fog was like. To start:

✔ Do a little research to find out which martial arts may appeal to you most.

✔ Make sure that you find a true master of the arts.

✔ Beware of anyone who claims that his particular style of martial arts is the one and only, who claims to know all the answers, or who demands an inordinate amount of your time and/or money. If anyone starts asking for your firstborn, it's a sure sign that you should bail out!

Strictly from a health standpoint, the soft, or internal, school of martial arts (like T'ai Chi) is generally considered more effective. The internal school of martial arts emphasizes the cultivation of qi (instead of brute force) and teaches you how to use your opponent's strength against him.

Then there's kickboxing, which has found adherents among women, and Tae Bo, which incorporates moves from martial arts for an aerobic workout — so it's not exactly a martial art per se. (Kickboxing and Tae Bo are considered hard forms.) Then, of course, you have your traditional martial arts from China, Japan, Korea, and other countries. Aside from T'ai Chi, other internal schools of martial arts include Hsing Yi and Bagua Zhang.

Chapter 9

All Stressed Out and Nowhere to Go

Have you been swinging high, swinging low, singing the blood sugar blues? Stress can do that to you. Ah, but don't get stressed-out over stress. Knowing how to handle stress can help you handle your hypoglycemia. This chapter provides hands-on info so you can relax and meditate.

How Stress Impacts Your Hypoglycemia

Stress can hinder attempts to balance your blood sugar level. When you're stressed, a series of biochemical changes takes place to prepare you to deal with your stressors: the old *fight-or-flight response*. When primitive man saw a saber-toothed tiger, he needed a burst of energy to fight or flee from the predator. Unless you're a big game hunter, you don't often run into hungry tigers or lions. Today, you're more likely to encounter threats in the form of job layoffs or work deadlines. But just like in the good ol' days of yore, the adrenal glands continue to pump you full of adrenaline so that you can either hightail it out of there or do battle. When you deal with stress day after day, your body begins to break down.

To compound the problem, many people turn to food when they're faced with continued stress. We sure don't need to tell you that most people aren't grabbing a celery stick or a bowl of steamed green beans to help themselves deal with stress. Alas, they use sugar as a quick pick-me-up. In response to the sugar, the body secretes too much insulin, as well as — guess what — more adrenaline! And the vicious cycle is perpetuated. This cycle is even more vicious if you happen to be hypoglycemic, because you already have a problem balancing your blood sugar.

Stress may cause, or at least exacerbate, the symptoms of low blood sugar. Some healthcare practitioners suspect that the body's inability to deal effectively with stress may be at the root of most manifestations of hypoglycemia. Some even believe that stress is one of the key factors, a hidden cause of not only hypoglycemia but also all diseases. Not enough studies have been done to conclusively support this hypothesis. But you don't need a whole lot of science to convince most people that too much stress just doesn't agree with their system.

Determining Your Stress Level

If you know you're already stressed, feel free to gloss over this section. You can jump to the remaining sections in this chapter that help you relax. Even if you're stressed, you may be tempted to skip this section because you think it's "only stress." After all, stress is no big deal; it's not like it's a disease or anything, right? Wrong. Stress is at the root of many illnesses. Even if it's not the direct cause of an ailment, it can be a contributing factor. At the very least it makes life worse, not better, and the road to recovery from an illness much rockier.

So if you can, we urge you to take a moment to discover how to de-stress and de-compress. The little bit of time you spend busting stress can pay dividends many times over.

Before you can discover how to relax your muscles, you need to recognize when and why they're tense. You can recognize the tension by consciously tuning in to your body. If you live primarily in your head, you're more likely to lend your ears to telemarketers than to your own body. Now you have a chance to get in touch with how your body feels.

Take the Life Stress Test, developed in 1997 by Dr. Tim Lowenstein to help determine how stressed you are, at www.cliving.org/ lifestresstest.htm. The test is similar to the Holmes Rahe Social Adjustment Rating Scale test, which you can find at: www.cop.ufl. edu/safezone/doty/dotyhome/wellness/HolRah.htm. This stress test is valid whether you have blood sugar imbalances or not. You'll notice that each life event has a number assigned to it, from a low of 10 to a high of 100. (Just add up the points for what you're experiencing in your life.)

Knotting Off: Relaxing Your Tight Muscles

Because stress can have an adverse effect on your body, figuring out how to handle and get rid of it is critical. The art of relaxation — and it truly is an art — is the key to healthy living. If you suffer from hypoglycemia (and even other health conditions), you can alleviate many hypoglycemic symptoms with proper relaxation techniques. If you're sugar-balance-challenged, you will find these techniques indispensable as you transition to a healthier diet. Making healthy changes doesn't have to be a grin-and-bear-it situation. If you use the methods outlined here and take the vitamins that help to curb any food cravings (see Chapter 7 for supplements and other natural remedies), you'll be able to make a smooth transition to a healthy lifestyle.

The following progressive muscle relaxation exercise helps you feel the difference between relaxed and tense muscles. It also helps you discover how to loosen up those tightly wound muscles. When performing this exercise, avoid overstraining yourself. Simply follow these instructions:

1. **Go somewhere quiet where you won't be disturbed.**

2. **Lie down on a bed (or wherever you can get comfortable).**

3. **Loosen any clothes that may be too tight.**

4. **Take a few breaths in and out.**

5. **Place your hand on your stomach and breathe in deeply while you press down.**

   Feel how your stomach expands when you breathe deeply.

6. **Tense your feet and curl your toes downward.**

   Hold for a few seconds and then release. Don't hold your breath. Breathe normally for the rest of the exercise.

7. **Tense your calves so that your toes are bent toward your face.**

   Don't tighten so much that you get cramps. Hold for a few seconds and then relax.

8. **Tighten your sphincter muscles (in the anal region).**

   Hold and release.

9. **Tighten your buttocks and thighs.**

   Hold and release. Feel the difference between tight and relaxed muscles.

10. **Clench your fists as you also tighten your forearms and upper arms.**

    Hold for a few seconds and then release.

11. **Shrug your shoulders and bring them up toward your ears.**

    Hold and release.

12. **Tighten your stomach.**

    Hold and release.

13. **Arch your back without straining.**

    Hold and release. Be very careful if you have a back problem.

14. **Open your mouth wide and feel the tension in your jaw and neck.**

    Be careful not to tense up too much, because you may hurt yourself. Hold for a few seconds and then relax. Your lips should be slightly parted.

15. **Squeeze your eyes closed tight and then relax.**

    Keep your eyes closed and feel the warmth spread across your eyelids.

16. **Raise your eyebrows as high as they will go so that your forehead gets wrinkled.**

    Hold and release. Smooth out your forehead completely.

17. **Tense your entire body.**

    Hold for several seconds and then release. Repeat this step two more times. When you're finished, you should feel a pleasant wave of relaxation sweep over you. All your muscles will feel loose and soft. Try to remember this sensation.

With this exercise, you feel how the sensations of tension and relaxation differ. It lets you know how you're supposed to feel when you're relaxed. As you keep practicing, inducing this state of relaxation becomes easier. For instance, assume that you agree to go out to eat with your friends even though you feel somewhat volatile. Then, someone suggests chipping in on a meal that's definitely off-limits for you. You don't want the situation to stress you out. You need to be able to take care of yourself without antagonizing anyone. What should you do? At times like this, you can do a mini-version of the muscle relaxation technique by tensing the muscles of your arms and legs and then releasing them. This shortened version will help diffuse any tension you may feel.

Although you may start noticing improvements almost immediately, it may be weeks or months before you're free of the physical and emotional problems associated with hypoglycemia. However, you can gain immediate relief by the progressive relaxation of your muscles. The relaxation exercises help with anxiety, depression, and fatigue, among other things, and unlike medication, they don't cause any negative side effects.

Taking a Deep Breath to Relax

Do you want a quick, fast stress fix? Something that will deliver an instant boost, get you turbocharged, and make you tingle with life and energy? Okay, then take a deep breath. And then another. There you have it: Breathing is the elixir of life. Breathing is something you can do at any time. And it costs absolutely nothing.

This section looks at how breathing can help your blood sugar. In this section, we also provide two breathing exercises — one for when you're in a hurry and another for when you have extra time to really inhale.

Breathing helps regulate your blood sugar

Breathing helps you become less irritated, less depressed, and less prone to such problems as panic attacks, anxiety, muscle tension, headaches, and fatigue (all of which are symptoms of hypoglycemia). That's right, deep breathing can help you alleviate many distressing symptoms and at the same time help regulate your blood sugar. It can also help you beat food addictions and food cravings.

People have attested to giving up all kinds of addictions, such as cigarette smoking and candy bars, just by deep breathing. Despite all the benefits gained from deep breathing, most people are underbreathers who are totally stingy about the way they breathe. (You'd think that they were being charged by the minute or the gallon.) Unless you're the exception, you probably suffer from a lack of serious breathing (especially if you have any health issues, including hypoglycemia).

In addition to your regular deep-breathing sessions, you should switch to your deep-breathing mode when you feel

- Dizzy
- Lightheaded

> ✔ Irritated
>
> ✔ Angry
>
> ✔ Anxious
>
> ✔ Fatigued
>
> ✔ Achy
>
> ✔ Cravings for sugar or simple starches (cakes, croissants, colas, fries, and so on)

Trying some deep-breathing exercises to relax

When you're stressing over daily problems, you may feel like you have no time to relax. Other times you may have an hour to wind down, but you're so worked up that you don't know how to take a chill pill. This section provides you with two deep breathing techniques.

The great thing about these breathing exercises is that they make you feel instantly revived. You'll get the most benefit, though, if you make these exercises a regular practice. After several months of these breathing exercises, you may even be able to blow down a brick house (although I wouldn't hold my breath waiting for that to happen). At the very least, your friends will be impressed by the dynamo that you've become. Just don't try deep breathing on the phone.

The quickie method

This technique is a handy-dandy way to perk you up anytime you're feeling dragged out. It can be a good way to start out the morning. Come to think of it, you may want to use it to end the day, too.

Just follow these easy steps on your way to stress relief:

1. **Inhale through your nose for a count of four to six (as many you can manage comfortably).**

2. **Hold the air in your lungs for a count of four to six.**

   Hold for the same number of counts as your inhalation. In other words, if you inhaled for a count of four, hold for a count of four.

3. **Exhale through your nose for a count of four to six.**

   If you inhaled for a count of four, exhale for a count of four.

Feel free to use this technique as much as you want. Are you sitting at a long traffic light and have two minutes? Waiting in the dentist's office before your appointment? Take a deep breath and relax.

The drawn-out method

When you have a bit more alone time, turn off your phone and television, and practice the following deep-breathing technique.

Plan to spend up to 20 minutes breathing in and out, and follow these steps for deep breathing:

1. **Lie down on a rug or exercise mat on the floor and bend your knees, keeping your feet about shoulder width apart.**

2. **Relax any areas of your body that are tight.**

   If you like, do the progressive muscle relaxation technique that we describe earlier in this chapter.

3. **Keep your mouth closed but relaxed.**

4. **Put one hand on your chest and the other on your stomach.**

5. **Breathe in deeply through your nose to the count of five.**

   Your abdomen should push up into your hand as much as possible. Your chest, however, should move only slightly. The hand on your chest will allow you to determine whether you're moving your chest too much.

6. **Exhale through your mouth.**

7. **Continue deep breathing for 5 to 20 minutes.**

Surfing the Alpha Wave with Meditation

Meditation occurs when you become relaxed and have a heightened sense of alertness. This effective antidote for stress and tension induces mental tranquility and physical relaxation, reduces high blood pressure, and improves circulation. Studies also show that meditating can boost the intensity of *alpha waves,* brain waves associated with quiet, receptive states of the mind that are conducive to relaxation and creativity.

For all you hyper-driven go-getters, rest assured that meditating isn't the same as vegetating. Nor does meditating have to be anything quaint or mystical — you don't have to sprout a beard and sit in the lotus position in front of a temple. Think of meditation as a way of focusing your mind on one thing. If you're confused, distracted, or anxious — all side effects of low blood sugar — meditation can help you to not only concentrate but also achieve serenity. Countless studies have shown the benefit of regular meditation in relieving stress and promoting good health. Meditation helps alleviate high blood pressure, heart disease, diabetes, arthritis, anxiety, depression, and so on. It can definitely aid you in regulating your blood sugar and anything else that's off kilter.

This section explains how you can use meditation in several different ways to relax, get energized, and even kick food cravings to the curb.

Balancing your blood and body

Some doctors suspect that the symptoms of hypoglycemia may be caused more by the release of stress hormones than by low blood sugar. If this theory is true, hypoglycemics should be able to drastically reduce the frequency and severity of their symptoms through the practice of meditation. It's been scientifically proven that meditating on a regular basis can relieve chronic pain, lower levels of stress hormones, and improve circulation.

A smorgasbord of meditations is out there for you to choose from. You can try Zen meditation, transcendental meditation, Tibetan Buddhist meditation, Taoist meditation, and insight meditation (also called Vipassana), to name just a few. Check out *Meditation For Dummies,* by Stephan Bodian (Wiley), for further information.

Starting with some simple oms

To start off, meditate for just five minutes a day. If you make meditation a habit, you'll be able to gradually go longer. Experienced practitioners meditate for an hour or even longer. Meditate for the amount of time that fits your schedule, but do make meditation a regular practice. The important thing is to meditate every day. As with anything, practice, patience, and persistence are what count the most.

Before you start meditating, turn off the TV, and if possible, put yourself in a room where you can close the door — and put up a "Do Not Disturb" sign. If you can't lock yourself in a room, do the best you can. Ask the people around you not to disturb you while you meditate. Meditating can be a bit tricky if you have small children. See if you can get a friendly neighbor to help you out. If not, try meditating for five minutes at a time.

Here's a simple meditation using a *mantra* (a type of incantation or affirmation):

1. **Sit in a chair or on the floor.**

   Sit wherever is most comfortable for you. Keep your back straight.

2. **Close your eyes, take a few deep breaths, relax, and try to quiet your mind.**

3. **Repeat the word *om* silently to yourself.**

   Or make up a hypo-specific mantra, such as "I'm becoming healthier." Don't worry if you keep having distracting thoughts. Just bring your awareness back to the mantra and continue repeating it. Try it for anywhere from 5 to 20 minutes.

4. **Take a few deep breaths and slowly open your eyes.**

You may be aware of a lot of thoughts during this meditation. You may even forget that you're supposed to be meditating. (Don't worry if you do; most people have that experience.) Through regular meditation practice, you can discover how to train the *monkey mind,* that unruly, undisciplined mind that flits from one thought to the next. When your mind chatter is turned down to a reasonable volume, you may find your mind becoming serene — more like the surface of a quiet lake rather than a turbulent stream.

Focusing on your breathing to meditate

If you don't like repeating words, you may want to try another basic meditation where you pay attention to your breathing. This meditation is great for toning the belly and helping relieve constipation. It's also a great way to relax before a test or an interview.

Here's a variation from a Taoist form of meditation:

1. **Sit in a chair or cross-legged on the floor.**

   Keep your back straight and your shoulders relaxed and sloping downward. Avoid jutting out your chin: It should be tucked in slightly, but not too much.

2. **Relax your jaw and lightly touch your tongue on the inside of your upper front teeth.**

3. **Close your eyes partially so that you're gazing softly downward, not focusing on anything.**

4. **Bring your attention to your *Dan Tien,* which is located inside your abdomen about an inch below your belly button.**

Think of the Dan Tien as your energy center, the cauldron in your belly. Dan Tien is the reservoir for your *qi,* or life force. You can read more about Dan Tien in *T'ai Chi For Dummies,* by Therese Iknoian (Wiley). There are other locations for the Dan Tien, but this spot suits the purposes of this exercise.

5. **Inhale deeply as you expand your abdomen.**

6. **Exhale as you contract your abdomen.**

Keep your attention lightly centered on the Dan Tien as you inhale and exhale.

Aside from your regular sessions, you can meditate whenever you experience any pain or discomfort from the side effects of low blood sugar. Meditation can help enormously as you change to healthier eating habits. It can help lessen your mood swings; the contrast between the hills and valleys that you experience won't be quite so sharp. If you find yourself going up and down emotionally, try meditation, breathing exercises, or progressive muscle relaxation. Or combine all three!

Energizing with EFT

One unusual way of beating stress — and hypoglycemia — is a nontraditional psychotherapy called Emotional Freedom Technique (EFT), also known as *meridian therapy,* or *energy medicine. EFT* is like acupuncture without needles. It helps calm your mind and balance your energy. It's one of the more popular forms of a healing modality based on energy medicine (see Chapter 4 for more on alternative medicine). Practitioners claim that EFT can provide quick relief from pain, diseases, and emotional issues.

Mental health professionals, alternative healthcare practitioners, and even some medical doctors are increasingly utilizing EFT. One reason EFT is becoming so popular is that it's fast, easy to learn, and you can do it on yourself.

What is EFT?

The term meridian therapy came about because EFT is based on the same energy meridians used in traditional Chinese medicine (TCM) to treat physical and emotional ailments. The premise is that meridians are connected to bodily organs and functions, and they act as channels through which the body's vital energy (*qi* or *chi*) circulates. Illnesses are caused by disruptions in this flow of qi. Blockages in the meridians act like dams that keep the river-water from nourishing the land it's flowing through. Traditional acupuncture attempts to treat illnesses by clearing such blocks and restoring energetic balance.

EFT works in a manner similar to acupuncture — it attempts to restore harmony by clearing energetic blockages. That's why EFT is sometimes described as *psychological acupuncture*. It brings the principles of acupuncture into the practice of psychotherapy by treating emotional as well as physical issues. But — and you'll be relieved to hear this — there are no needles involved. All that's necessary are your fingertips for tapping on the various meridian points.

EFT practitioners believe that unresolved negative emotions are the major contributors to most physical pains and diseases. Negative emotions impede and disrupt the body's qi. Because the emotions are connected to physical pains and diseases, when you clear them out, the corresponding physical illness or discomfort is gone.

Using EFT to relax

According to EFT founder Gary Craig, clearing negative emotions and residues of emotional trauma by digging into unresolved issues from childhood may allow the body to heal itself. The body will then become effective at maintaining a good blood sugar balance. The individual may even find that foods that used to put the body into a tailspin no longer cause problems. (This doesn't, of course, negate the importance of eating a proper diet; it just means that you have a little more leeway about what you do or don't eat.)

EFT can also be used to reduce or eliminate any of the symptoms of hypoglycemia, such as headaches and dizziness. Follow these steps to try EFT treatment:

1. **Focus on a disturbing memory, emotion, or specific issue (such as a traumatic event or addiction).**

   You can use EFT also on specific hypoglycemic symptoms such as dizziness, headaches, irritability, and so forth. If there are emotional issues you believe may be triggering your symptoms, you can address them with EFT.

   This exercise is supposed to remove the emotional block from the body's energy system, thus restoring it to harmony and balance. This restoration then helps heal the physical disease.

2. **Start with a setup phrase that sets the stage for an EFT treatment.**

   For example, if you're trying to work on a hypoglycemic symptom such as a headache, the setup phrase may go something like this: "Even though I have a headache (or I have a deep/dull/throbbing pain in the right/left/front/back side of my head), I deeply and completely love and accept myself."

   Apply this phrase to the specific event, emotion, or condition in question. Make an attempt to accept that experience and reaffirm love and acceptance of yourself. You don't have to believe the setup phrase or subsequent statements for EFT to work.

3. **Repeat the setup phrase and tap the "karate chop" meridian point at the side of the hand (see Figure 9-1).**

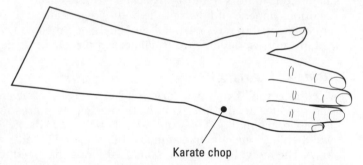

Karate chop

Figure 9-1: Use the area outside the hand to deliver light karate taps.

4. **Tap the following points (see Figure 9-2) using the *reminder phrase,* which keeps your mind and body tuned into the issue that you're addressing:**

   - Top of the head (H)

   - Toward the inside of the eyebrows and slightly above them (EB)

   - Outside corner of the eyes, on the side (SE)

   - On opposite sides of the face; under the center of the eyes (UE)

   - Midway between the nose and the upper lip (UN)

   - Midway between the lower lip and the chin (CH)

- Two points at the beginning of the collarbone at the edge where it meets the breastbone (CB)

- Under the arms, about three to four inches below the armpit, roughly level with the chest (UA)

You can tap three or more times on each point. There are no hard and fast rules about this. There are a few other points as well, but these are the most commonly used. An example of a reminder phrase (if you're working on a headache) is "This headache (or this dull pain in the side of my head — or whatever is true about what you're experiencing)."

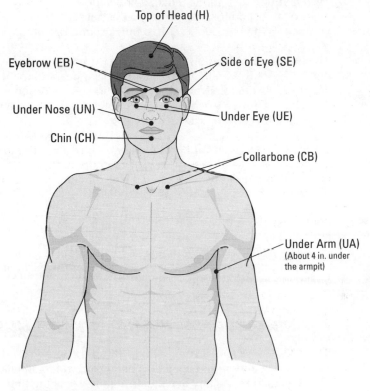

Figure 9-2: Tap these meridian points.

Identifying the pros and cons of using EFT

You can try EFT on any hypoglycemic symptom. But make sure you're eating at regular intervals. And, if you're a diabetic who experiences a sudden drop in blood sugar, you must follow your doctor's instructions on dealing with such emergencies. This may mean taking glucose tablets or drinking orange juice to quickly raise the blood sugar.

The following are advantages of EFT:

- ✔ Easy to learn
- ✔ Simple to use
- ✔ Quick
- ✔ Requires no special equipment
- ✔ You can do it anywhere
- ✔ Takes only a few minutes

Even if you're in a public place, if you suddenly feel any physical or emotional discomforts, or simply feel stressed, you can excuse yourself to the bathroom to do a quick round or two of tapping.

The biggest disadvantage of EFT is that as a healing technique, it's currently controversial. A few studies have been done, but nothing conclusively demonstrates that EFT works as its proponents claim. All evidence for EFT benefits is anecdotal. No one has reported any adverse effects from EFT.

Using EFT effectively and proficiently requires additional study; watch DVDs, take a class or two, or read up on the subject. We urge you to check out Gary Craig's Web site at www.emofree.com to discover how to use EFT properly.

If you suspect that you may be suffering from symptoms of chronic hypoglycemia, always consult your physician and get a thorough medical checkup before choosing a further course of action. Never attempt to diagnose or treat yourself without the assistance of a qualified medical practitioner.

Kicking food cravings in the gut

Because stress can trigger cravings for all the wrong foods — sugar, sugar, and more sugar! — meditation, which alleviates stress, can be especially beneficial. So are stress-busting exercises like yoga and T'ai Chi. Just practicing them may help cut down on your cravings. (See Chapter 8 for more info on yoga and T'ai Chi.)

Meditating away your cravings

As you develop mindfulness with meditation, you become more aware of your eating habits. As much as people may be obsessed with food, most don't pay sufficient attention to what they're eating. In fact, many people seem to go almost unconscious when they eat.

To become more conscious about your eating, try the following meditation:

1. **Pick a time when you're home alone.**

   If you live with people, do the meditation in your room or somewhere you can have privacy, and ask everyone not to disturb you.

2. **Place the food in front of you.**

   This can be any food (good, bad, or indifferent) that you're about to eat. The object is to become more aware of what you're eating.

3. **Take several deep breaths.**

4. **Note the color, shape, and texture of the food.**

   - **Note any reactions you have.** How do you feel about the food? Does it look appealing to you?

   - **Notice how your body reacts to the food.** What physical sensations do you have?

5. **Now bring the food to your mouth.**

   - **Smell the food.** What is your reaction to the smell?

   - **Take a bite.** How does it feel to bite into the food?

   - **Chew the food.** How does the food feel to your lips, teeth, and tongue? What other sensations do you notice?

   - **As you swallow the food, pay attention to how your esophagus contracts and relaxes.** Can you feel the food traveling down to your stomach?

   - **Note how your stomach feels after you swallow the food.**

6. **Put the food down between bites and breathe deeply.**

7. **Take another bite.**

   Again, pay attention to all the sensations.

This meditation helps you become more conscious of the act of eating. You can also try this meditation when you're eating a forbidden food. Rather than cram your food down in a rush or with a feeling of guilt, be as fully conscious as you can when you eat. And enjoy what you're eating! If paying attention to all the details gets tedious after awhile, just remain focused on the taste and smell of the food, and relish it as much as you can.

Using EFT to fight food cravings

Many people report that with the help of EFT, they've been able to reduce or eliminate cravings for sugar and other food. (Check out "Energizing with EFT" earlier in this chapter for more info about EFT.)

Consider the following when trying EFT with food cravings:

1. **Judge the intensity of the craving, using a simple scale of 0 to 10.**

   On this scale, 0 means least intense and 10 most intense.

2. **Follow the steps that we describe in "Using EFT to relax," earlier in this chapter.**

3. **While tapping the karate chop meridian point, say the following to yourself as a setup phrase:**

   • Even though I'm really craving this piece of cake and I want to take a bite right now, I deeply and completely love and accept myself.

4. **Tap the sequence of meridian points, and repeat a reminder phrase to yourself, such as:**

   • Craving this cake. (Choose any reminder phrase that works well for you, such as "I really want to eat this," "I desire this cake intensely," or "I really need this cake!")

   You may think that repeating a phrase like this will only intensify the craving. In fact, by stating the truth of how you're feeling at the moment, you help to release it.

5. **Rate the intensity of the craving again.**

   Is it less intense? Is it completely gone? Repeat the tapping sequence until you no longer crave the food.

You can make up your own setup and reminder phrases according to your own needs and your own situation. Do whatever works best for you. For best results, combine EFT with other techniques for reducing or eliminating food cravings. (Check out Chapter 16 for some additional self-help hints.)

Making the Ultimate Smoothie: Hypno-Soothing

Self-hypnosis is another tool you can use if you hit rough patches in your effort to transition to a hypoglycemic diet. You can use it to

help stick to your food plan or alleviate uncomfortable hypoglycemic symptoms.

Don't be spooked by the word *hypnosis*. It's not witchcraft, and it's
not a séance. And you won't be clucking around like a hen either,
because self-hypnosis isn't the same as stage hypnosis, where the
focus is on showmanship rather than healing. You can find it very
relaxing, in fact. With self-hypnosis, you're the one in charge. You
maintain total control. It's not dangerous, and you can do it alone.

You can hypnotize yourself in many different ways. Here's one
simple method:

1. **Pick a quiet time and place where you won't be disturbed.**

2. **Play soothing music if you think that it may help you,
   especially if background noise is a problem.**

3. **Lie down where you can be comfortable.**

   If you find that you keep falling asleep when you try to hypnotize yourself, sit in a chair.

4. **Inhale slowly and deeply.**

   Hold your breath and exhale slowly. Each time you exhale,
   imagine that you're releasing all your tension.

5. **Use the progressive muscle relaxation technique
   described in "Knotting off: Relaxing Your Tight Muscles"
   earlier in this chapter to help release all your tensions.**

   Work from your toes up, relaxing each muscle group.

6. **If your neck is stiff, do a few slow head rolls and really
   work to get your muscles relaxed.**

7. **Take as much time as you need to get fully relaxed.**

   It will take longer in the beginning, but later you'll achieve
   relaxation quickly.

8. **Imagine that you're in an elevator.**

   The floor indicator shows that you're on the 50th floor. The
   elevator begins to go down at a steady pace, not too fast, not
   too slow. You're on the 49th floor, and you're going down,
   down, down. Continue breathing deeply and slowly as you
   watch the numbers go down . . . 48th, 47th, and so on.

   If thoughts or other images intrude, just gently brush them
   aside.

   With each breath, you're going deeper and deeper.

9. **When the elevator arrives at the first floor, you're ready to give yourself suggestions.**

10. **You should now give yourself autosuggestions.**

Autosuggestions are statements that you repeat while in a hypnotic state to influence your own attitudes and behavior. Use words and statements that make sense to you, because they'll be more effective.

For example, you can say, "I naturally gravitate toward healthy foods," or "I'm finding it easier and easier to eat a healthy diet with plenty of fresh vegetables and fruits," or "I can now easily pass up processed foods that are filled with sugar and starch."

You can also make up statements to help ease your symptoms, such as, "I am now happy and emotionally balanced, and I'm becoming more and more energetic each day."

Make all your statements affirmative and in the present tense. Don't say, "I will not eat dessert anymore." Instead try, "I no longer have a desire for desserts that are full of sugar."

After you make your suggestion, you're ready to terminate the session.

11. **Terminate your session by counting to three.**

Say, "I'm going to count from one to three. At the count of three, I'll be totally refreshed, wide awake, and completely alert. One — I'm beginning to come out of it. Two — I'm coming out more, ready to wake up. Three — I'm wide awake, feeling refreshed and revitalized."

As with anything, you need to set up a regular time of practice, and you need to do it consistently, or you won't get the results you want. You won't get instant results, but you should start to see some changes in a few weeks. If you don't notice changes during this time, examine your suggestions and try different ones. If you feel you need more support and advice on what to do, consider trying one of the numerous books and tapes on self-hypnosis. However, the information outlined here should be enough to get you going.

Chapter 10

Defanging the Depression Demons

. . . .

In This Chapter

▶ Recognizing symptoms of depression

▶ Discovering how neurotransmitters function

▶ Checking out the different types of therapy

▶ Treating your condition with antidepressants

. . . .

*W*atch out for the demons of depression. If you have chronic problems with low blood sugar, they're sure to attack you sooner or later. Of course, they're not real demons with horns and fangs. In a way, though, these demons are much more frightening, because they're invisible and they attack one of your most vulnerable areas — your state of mind.

Why is depression one of hypoglycemia's main symptoms? Because its sisters — anxiety, irritability, poor concentration, feelings of panic, and suicidal tendencies — are just a few things hypoglycemia can create. Hypoglycemics also tend to suffer from temper tantrums, mood swings, and crying jags. (See Chapter 3 for more symptom info.) These symptoms aren't surprising, considering that the brain uses glucose as its fuel. When you don't have enough glucose circulating in your blood, your brain begins to starve. At rest, the brain consumes a third of the body's total glucose requirement.

This chapter sheds light on how to deal with stresses that may be keeping you hooked to the hypoglycemic cycle of eating the wrong foods, making you feel even sicker and causing you to reach for foods that trigger bouts of hypoglycemia . . . and on and on.

Revealing Another Epidemic

According to the National Institute of Mental Health (NIMH), an estimated 6.7 million people in established market economies, such as the United States, suffer from depression. That's 6.8 percent of the population. In fact, major depression (not just your ordinary everyday blues, but a serious medical condition) is the leading cause of disability worldwide. These statistics may seem misleading, because many people are unaware of their depression, and others resist seeking proper treatment. Depression still tends to be regarded as a character defect or a weakness of will rather than as a multifaceted illness.

Depression is not only the most undertreated medical illness, but also the most treatable. Treatment is said to be effective in more than 80 percent of cases. Perhaps most of the cases that have been resistant to treatment can be affected through proper dietary changes.

To help you recognize the symptoms of depression in yourself and others, here are some questions adapted from the National Institutes of Health:

- Are you persistently sad?
- Do you feel "empty" most of the time, and do you feel that life is meaningless?
- Has your energy decreased lately? Do you feel tired most of the time?
- Do you no longer find pleasure in activities you used to enjoy, including sex?
- Have you been experiencing sleep disturbances? Is it hard for you to sleep? Do you wake up in the middle of the night or early in the morning? Do you oversleep?
- Have you recently lost or gained a lot of weight? Have you lost your appetite? Do you overeat?
- Do you suffer from feelings of guilt, worthlessness, or helplessness?
- Have you been feeling more irritable than usual?
- Do you cry frequently?
- Do you have chronic aches and pains that don't respond to medical treatment?
- Do you have thoughts of death or suicide? Have you made any suicide attempts?

But how does sugar make you feel?

People often show affection and reward others by offering sugary treats. In most Western cultures (and other cultures, as well), sugar has become its own reward system. People have become conditioned to crave gooey desserts. As a result, so many emotional issues (not to mention excess weight) revolve around excess sugar consumption.

Sugar, therefore, can become a compulsive habit. For some, it becomes a true addiction. (To read more about sugar and addiction, flip to Chapter 2.) You know if you're an addict. Your friends may be able to eat a few cookies and leave the rest; get a few scoops of ice cream without devouring the entire tub; or eat just one square of a chocolate bar. But you? If you're a sugar junkie, you know what you do. And it's not pretty. If you're addicted to sugar, you may need to completely abstain from the substance, at least temporarily, to free yourself from your addiction. No matter what's causing your craving for sugar, you may be able to meet it by eating fruits or an occasional natural dessert made without refined sugar.

If you answer yes to the last question, immediately call 911, a suicide prevention hotline (whose number should be in the yellow pages), or your company's confidential employee assistance program. You also need to call if you think that someone else is considering suicide.

In addition, you may have difficulty remembering, concentrating, or making decisions. You may engage in destructive self-criticism or experience low self-esteem, and you may abuse drugs or alcohol. Bear in mind that these are all hallmarks of low blood sugar. Many unwitting sufferers become *substance addicts* in an unconscious effort to medicate themselves.

If you've had five or more of these symptoms for two weeks or longer, you may be suffering from depression. You owe it to yourself to seek professional help.

Knowing What (Gray) Matters

The brain is that gray matter people so-matter-of-factly take for granted. Brain cells, or *neurons,* communicate by releasing a chemical called a *neurotransmitter.* To put it simply, your moods change in response to the fluctuating levels of these neurotransmitters.

A deficiency or imbalance in any of these transmitters can cause problems such as depression, sleeplessness, and irritability. It's believed that a deficiency or imbalance of these neurotransmitters is the underlying cause of depression. As you can see from Table 10-1, many neurotransmitters perform various functions.

Table 10-1 Some Neurotransmitters and Their Functions	
Major Neurotransmitters	*Some of Their Functions*
Endorphins	Elevate mood; act as a natural pain killer; produce loving feelings
Norepinephrine	Improves alertness; produces feelings of excitement and happiness; appetite control
Dopamine	Produces feelings of pleasure and euphoria; appetite control
Acetylcholine	Improves alertness, memory, and sexual performance
Phenylethylmine	Produces feelings of bliss and infatuation (Chocolate is a lover's delight because of its high levels of phenylethylmine!)
Serotonin	Relieves depression; diminishes cravings; improves self-confidence and impulse control

Getting Comfy on the Couch

Are you troubled, stressed, or depressed? If so, you may benefit from *psychotherapy* — therapy of the mind and emotions. *Psychotherapists,* professionals who administer psychotherapy, can help you find healthier ways to relate to others and unlearn behavior that leads to unwanted consequences.

Would you like some yin with your coffee?

From the point of view of traditional Chinese medicine, the desire for sweet flavor is seen as a craving for comfort and security, and a longing for the mother, which is a *yin* energy. Yin represents dark, female, cold, the earth, and so on. Its opposite, *yang,* is regarded as light, male, warm, and heaven. The stressful urban setting is seen as having a yang energy, and city dwellers may unconsciously seek to balance the excessive yang by turning to sweets and starches, which are yin.

If your depression is mainly a result of blood sugar imbalance, you may find that no amount of talk therapy can keep the beast at bay until the underlying disorder is corrected. So don't use therapy as an excuse to shirk your diet. A healthy diet and therapy work hand-in-hand. Even if you choose not to see a therapist today, a plethora of self-help techniques can help you deal with mood disorders. Meditation, relaxation and progressive techniques, stress-management, and self-hypnosis mean that you'll never be bored. See Chapter 9 for more information about these subjects.

If you do want to tackle bad habits that stem from hypoglycemia's physical causes (such as sugar addiction), or if you just want to get yourself out of that funky depression (such as the one making you cry every other day), therapy may benefit you. To pick a good therapist, refer to Chapter 4; the suggestions for hooking up with the right doctor apply to therapists, as well.

This section sheds some light on what therapy can do to battle your depression. This section also explains how a therapist can help you start thinking in a healthy manner.

Mastering new thinking skills

After years of suffering from low blood sugar, you or your loved one may have fallen into the habit of distorted, negative thinking. You may worry too much, anticipate the worst, discount your achievements, get offended easily, and so on. You may feel as though you have no control over your feelings.

The good news is that anyone can discover how to replace damaging thoughts with more positive and realistic thoughts. When you tackle these counterproductive thoughts, it becomes easier to choose a lifestyle that supports your goals of maximum health and happiness.

What can therapists do for you to help you battle your depression? They can:

- ✔ **Teach you new ways of thinking and of looking at things by questioning your assumptions and pointing out the thoughts that lead to feelings of anxiety, depression, or other negatives.** If you're like most people, you have a tendency to believe all your thoughts. In other words, you accept your beliefs as self-evident truths — when in fact, they're nothing more than assumptions that you've made about yourself or your life. For example, if you're depressed, you may tell yourself, "It's just the way things are; my symptoms are here to stay." "Learning how to eat a hypoglycemically correct diet is too daunting a task. I can never do it." These are unquestioned assumptions that can keep you from recovering from your health condition — or attaining any other cherished desires.

✔ **Help you regain control over your feelings by teaching you how to define and set goals, and how to take small, incremental steps toward achieving them.** After you discover how to break your goals into small steps, you'll find it easier to make steady progress.

✔ **Help you deal better with hypoglycemic symptoms and tolerate the physical aches that are hypoglycemia's hallmark.** At the same time, therapy can teach you to become more consistent at treating the disorder (for instance, by eating better and learning to incorporate exercise into your life). Ups and downs are inevitable while you're transitioning to a healthier lifestyle, and the support of a good therapist can be indispensable. *Psychology For Dummies,* by Adam Cash, PsyD (Wiley), discusses the various types of therapy and takes on tough therapy topics. Read it for more in-depth information.

If you don't want to see a therapist, you may want to start with self-help books. Books on changing your *cognitive patterns* can also be very helpful. Negative patterns of thinking feed depression. For instance, if you persistently think, "I'm a failure. There's nothing I can do to help myself," you're bound to feel helpless and hopeless. When you change these negative, habitual ways of thinking, you lift your mood. This is a useful therapy to try if you've been living with hypoglycemia and all its distorted thinking. Check out your local library or bookstore for good titles on the subject. Get books that guide you through changing your negative thoughts, step by step, and provide concrete examples.

Thinking healthy

According to a controlled study by the University of Pennsylvania, people who maintain optimistic attitudes not only avoid depression but also improve their physical health. When students were taught *cognitive coping skills,* they reported fewer physical problems. In other words, they replaced self-defeating thoughts ("I'm too stupid to get good grades") with more positive ones ("I'm intelligent and can get good grades if I apply myself").

Similar coping skills can be applied to hypoglycemia. For instance, you may find yourself thinking, "How come everyone else gets to have fun eating whatever, while I have to restrict my diet? And I'm not even noticing any improvement." Not only are these thoughts negative, they're generally not even true. These are all examples of distorted thinking. Some reflection will tell you that these thoughts don't accurately describe reality. They're unhelpful and can keep you stuck in unhealthy patterns of behavior.

Does your life coach wear a whistle?

One alternative to therapy is to hire a life coach. A *life coach* acts like a personal trainer for your life. Athletes have coaches who train, motivate, and help them perform, so why shouldn't you have a coach to assist you in designing and creating a better life? Life coaches can help you set goals, teach you necessary skills, and keep you on track. Consultations are available in person, by phone, or by e-mail. Just as with therapists, you need to carefully screen potential coaches. Because life coaches aren't required to undergo as rigorous a training program as psychotherapists, you need to be extra careful that you hire a person of integrity who can effectively guide you. Personal recommendations are probably the best.

Bear in mind that although coaches are supposed to honor confidentiality, they have no medical training, and they can't prescribe meds. Like sports coaches, they're good at motivating clients, but if you're currently suffering from depression, they'll be the first ones to tell you to see a licensed psychotherapist.

You can discover how to challenge your thoughts and identify what's irrational or unhelpful about them. When you spot the distortions, replace them with more realistic and more positive alternative thoughts. "If it's fun I want, there's lots I can do. Besides, I'm getting fewer headaches, and my mood swings aren't as severe. Even though I miss my favorite foods, becoming healthier is worth giving up bad habits." From this example, you can see how easily you can discourage — or encourage — yourself.

Like any new skill, it may take you awhile to get the hang of replacing negative thoughts with positive thoughts. You wouldn't expect to win a black belt overnight if you were learning judo. Be just as patient with yourself when you're learning to think healthy.

You also have the option of finding a psychotherapist trained in cognitive therapy or cognitive behavior therapy to help you if you find yourself struggling to master these new skills. The therapist can help you recognize destructive patterns of thinking and reacting, and then provide you with tools to help you modify or correct these errors.

Easing through the transition

When you've tackled counterproductive thoughts, it's easier to choose a lifestyle that supports your goals. A faulty body chemistry makes it difficult to make rational choices. If your battle with blood sugar imbalance has left you tired and weary, you can regain control by learning how to define and set goals and take small, incremental steps toward achieving them. If you don't know how to do this, read a book, take a course in goal-setting, or find a therapist who can help you define your goals.

Transitions can be difficult. One big plus about going on a recovery program for low blood sugar is that you start feeling so much better, and hence you're motivated to keep going. Of course, you may have setbacks and *plateaus* (when things stay the same and nothing seems to be happening), but if you honestly follow the food and exercise program, your symptoms will start disappearing, and you'll feel healthier.

This is where competent therapists can play a vital role. They teach you cognitive skills that you can use to address your transition. Also, you'll regain a sense of optimism knowing that you're tackling your problem head-on with a compassionate professional on your side.

Beating the Low Blood Sugar Blues

The best way out of the low blood sugar blues is simple — right through your mouth. (We don't mean singing, but you can try that, too.) You can eat your way to hell or health, your choice. If you truly want to beat the blues, start by looking at how your diet affects your mood when you have hypoglycemia. You can then make the necessary dietary changes to help battle the blues. (Chapter 6 focuses on actual dietary changes; this section focuses on the relationship of your diet and depression and how you can overcome that depression.)

Stop being so SAD

The sort of food that most Americans — and increasingly, the rest of the world — consume is called SAD (Standard American Diet) for a good reason. Stick with it long enough and you're likely to start feeling sad and depressed. Why? The diet consists of too much refined sugar and refined flour, has tons of hydrogenated oil and other bad oils, and is high in calories and low in nutrients. Now, if that doesn't depress you, what would! If scientists went to their labs to deliberately cook up (no pun intended) a diet designed to cause blood sugar imbalance, they couldn't come up with a better — or rather, worse — diet than this one.

Sadly, SAD appears to have ignited an epidemic of diabetes in the United States — and the rest of the world is following America's sad lead. Today, more than 20 million adults and children in the United States have diabetes.

So how does this relate to hypoglycemia? Oddly enough, chronic problems with low blood sugar can lead to its opposite — high blood sugar, or type 2 diabetes. (Check out Chapter 3 for more info.) The underlying cause of both type 2 diabetes and hypoglycemia is poor nutrition. Poor diet leads to blood sugar imbalances. Unbalanced blood sugar can ravage your health and cause depression. (Check out Chapter 6 for ways to improve your diet.)

By some estimates, the incidence of major depression has increased tenfold since a decade ago. That's not too surprising, considering that there seems to be a hidden link between diabetes and depression. If you consider that one of the symptoms of hypoglycemia is depression, you can see how some depressed people may be prone to developing diabetes. It also makes sense that individuals suffering from a chronic disease like diabetes would have a tendency to become depressed. Research suggests that diabetes increases the risk of depression, and depression increases the risk of diabetes. It's not quite clear which comes first, diabetes or depression. But it really doesn't matter which comes first. What doctors are most concerned about is that depression interferes with an individual's problem-solving ability and therefore his ability to manage diabetes.

Taking a swing at your mood

The same drugs that treat clinical depression can also help with mood swings, one of the key symptoms of hypoglycemia. When your blood sugar is erratic — rising fast in response to eating, and then dropping too low shortly after — your moods are likely to swing wildly too. Antidepressants may work to stabilize your mood. (Check out the section "Feeling Out Antidepressants" for more info.) But each individual is different, and a drug that works for one person may not necessarily work for another.

A more natural approach using herbs and supplements may work just as well as antidepressants, and without their side effects. (Chapter 7 tells you more about this subject.) Because each person's biochemistry is different, try to find a healthcare provider knowledgeable about hypoglycemia and depression to give you suggestions.

So many factors are involved in depression that it's too simplistic to say that poor diet is its only cause. Nonetheless, evidence has been mounting that depression and mood swings are linked to vitamin and mineral deficiencies. The following can help you keep your mood from swinging:

✔ **Obtain more Omega-3 fatty acids.** Good food sources are walnuts, flaxseed, and oily fish like salmon. But if you're fighting depression, start out by taking Omega-3 supplements in the form of fish oil capsules. (For resources on high-quality supplements, flip to Chapter 7.)

Here's an added bonus: Unlike antidepressants that often lead to decreased sex drive or the inability to experience orgasms, Omega-3s appear to help boost sex drive.

✔ **Get more folic acid.** Cabbage is rich in folic acid — or *folate,* when it occurs naturally in foods. It also has vitamin C and lots of fiber, which slows down digestion and stabilizes blood sugar. You can also take folic acid supplements.

✔ **Get plenty of natural sunlight.** Doing so can also help offset mood swings. If you live in an area without adequate sunshine, try full-spectrum light bulbs in your house.

✔ **Stay away from caffeine and tobacco smoke.** Both substances contribute to blood sugar imbalance.

✔ **Know about potential prescription drug side effects.** Some prescription medication, such as amphetamines, pain killers, anticonvulsants, high blood pressure drugs, and so forth, can also contribute to depression. But don't quit taking them or cut back on the dosage by yourself. Go talk to your doctor and see whether he can recommend alternative approaches.

Discussing dietary plans

No matter what you do, if hypoglycemia is the root cause of your depression or cravings, you have to change your diet — no way around that! It doesn't matter if you try talk therapy; over the long haul, not much can change unless you revamp your diet.

For instance, a woman in her 40s sought help from various therapists because she'd suffered from depression all her life. The therapists were able to help clear up many long-standing problems, but the depression didn't budge. Finally, they discovered that she had low blood sugar. When she changed her eating habits, her dark moods promptly went away.

For quick help in balancing your blood sugar, try some of these tips:

✔ **Replace simple carbs like white bread and white rice with complex starches.** For instance, brown rice has the following:

- More complex molecules that take longer for the body to digest (helping you avoid the sugar-insulin spike).

- Vitamins B1, B3, and folic acid to help prevent mood swings.

✔ **Eat whole grains like kamut, spelt, and quinoa, which contain nutrients beneficial to the brain.** Kamut contains more protein and amino acids than common wheat. Spelt has more vitamins B1 and B2 than other grains, and is also rich in magnesium and iron. Quinoa provides complete protein because it contains all eight essential amino aids. It's considered the best source of protein in the vegetable kingdom.

✔ **Plan healthy snacks.** Brazil nuts are easy to carry around when you're on the move and need a quick snack. Aside from being tasty, they're high in selenium, which may help in counteracting depression.

Some of the older antidepressants can increase sugar cravings, so tell your doctor that you need to avoid sweets. The newer antidepressant drugs don't have this side effect.

Going online to fight your depression

Are you battling some depression or anxiety? Do you feel blue or down in the dumps? If you're looking for additional help to deal with your depression and hypoglycemia, check out the following Web sites:

✔ **All of Depression (www.allofdepression.com):** This comprehensive Web site offers a directory, articles, and resources on depression.

✔ **The Anxiety & Hypoglycemia Relief Institute:** This group was founded by Professor J.H. Levitt in 1994. The group's purpose is to help educate people about the most common causes of biochemical imbalance. For questions regarding anxiety and hypoglycemia and New York City classes, contact Prof. Levitt at 212-479-7805 (voice mail) or jlevitt@pratt.edu (e-mail).

✔ **Health Recovery Center (www.healthrecovery.com):** This center was founded in 1980 by Joan Matthews Larson, PhD, author of *Seven Weeks to Sobriety.* Larson's article explains the link between hypoglycemia and alcoholism. This site provides comprehensive information about alcoholism, depression, and anxiety, and biochemical solutions to overcome them. It offers nutritional supplements suggested in her books, including a hypoglycemia formula. To contact this organization, phone 800-554-9155 or e-mail hrc@healthrecovery.com.

✔ **International Guide to the World of Alternative Mental Health (www.alternativementalhealth.com):** This site advocates non-drug approaches to mental health on the premise that underlying much of what are commonly regarded as mental disorders are allergies, nutritional imbalances, poor diets, lack of exercise, and other treatable physical conditions. It offers more than 100 articles, testimonials, a comprehensive directory of alternative mental health practitioners, support groups, e-mail lists, a free monthly newsletter, and a bookstore.

Feeling Out Antidepressants

The hypoglycemic diet is your first and best line of offense for low blood sugar. (Chapter 6 starts you on that journey.) Exercise, discussed in Chapter 8, is your next best bet. Following that, your mental health is the place to focus.

Serotonin deficiency, a condition where the brain isn't producing enough of the neurotransmitter serotonin, responsible for feelings of well-being, is correlated with depression, low self-esteem, sleep problems, worry, and irritability. A wide range of medications called *antidepressants* are used to treat clinical depression. These meds have varying effects on serotonin, norepinephrine, and dopamine. These same drugs help not only with depression but also with mood swings and some obsessive-compulsive disorders.

If your dark moods are caused by underlying metabolic disorders, antidepressants can generally work to stabilize your moods until you start making progress with your new food plan. You should be aware that when it comes to hypoglycemia, medication is not a substitute for the correct diet. Taking antidepressants without treating the underlying disorder that causes it is like banging your head against the wall while taking pain medication to relieve the headache. Sure, the drug will help, but shouldn't you stop hitting yourself?

This section takes a closer look at the different antidepressants available today and important pointers you need to remember if you're considering taking antidepressants.

Identifying the different drugs

Your psychiatrist can determine whether your depression may benefit from antidepressants, as well as the type of medication and dosage you need. (Psychologists aren't licensed to prescribe medications, so if you're seeing such a doctor, she may team up with a psychiatrist to make sure that you get the prescription you need.) Table 10-2 lists some common antidepressants. New drugs are continually developed and tested; your doctor can give you the latest information.

Table 10-2

Common Antidepressants

Pharmacological Name	Brand Names	How It Works	Pros	Cons
SSRI (Selective Serotonin Reuptake Inhibitors)	Zoloft, Prozac, Luvox, Paxil, Effexor, Celexa, Lexapro	Stabilizes serotonin levels.	They reportedly have fewer side effects, and no withdrawal symptoms. Thus, they're generally the first choice of most physicians.	Some media reports have implicated Prozac with mood disturbances and violent behavior, but evidence remains inconclusive. Drug can be transferred in breast milk.
TCA (Tricyclic Antidepressants)	Adapin, Endep, Norpramin, Pamelor, Sinequan	Thought to increase the brain's levels of norepinephrine, a neurotransmitter.	May be more effective for some patients.	Can cause heat sensitivity. Can cause the body to have difficulty adapting to temperature changes. Must be discontinued slowly, or withdrawal symptoms may occur.
MAOI (Monoamine Oxidase Inhibitors)	Nardil, Parnate	Increases levels of epinephrine, norepinephrine, and serotonin in the brain.	May be effective in cases where patient fails to respond to other medications.	Must adhere to a strict dietary regime: Failure to do so can be fatal. Many other medications react badly with MAOIs.

Bear in mind that relief may not come immediately. You may get lucky and, right off the bat, find what works for you. If not, you may need to go through a trial-and-error period before settling on the right medication and dosage. This process may take a month or longer. (To view a complete list of antidepressants, go to `www.fda.gov/cder/drug/antidepressants/MDD_all-druglist.pdf`.)

Mixing and matching clothes is fun, but you definitely don't want to recklessly combine drugs. Drugs and herbs can have serious interactions with other medications. Tell your doctor about anything you're taking, including vitamins, herbs, and supplements. Remember: Combination lunches may be an option in Chinese restaurants, but don't combine prescriptions without asking your doctor! As an example, avoid taking SSRI antidepressants (such as Prozac and Effexor) if you're also taking drugs for migraine headaches known as 5-hydroxytryptamine receptor agnoists (triptans). Taking these medicines together can sometimes result in *serotonin syndrome,* a condition leading to serious changes in the workings of your brain, muscles, and digestive system that can sometimes be fatal.

Considering antidepressants? Know both sides of the story

Although pharmaceutical companies heavily promote antidepressants, these drugs have multiple side effects, and the long-term effects on the brain and body haven't yet been fully evaluated. It's too soon to say with certainty that the most popular *psychotropic drugs* (drugs that act on your mind) on the market today are completely safe over the long haul. A debate has been raging over the safety and efficacy of these drugs.

The good

Never take any drugs for trivial reasons. Thousands of people have tried antidepressants without major side effects when taken as prescribed. Many report that the medication has helped lift them out of their melancholy and given them a new lease on life. One patient compared antidepressants to "a splint for a broken spirit," while another likened them to wings that allowed her to fly.

Even if you get so chummy with your family physician that you lose all respect for the poor doc, you should never, ever lose respect for antidepressants. They must be treated with caution, if not reverence. Be careful about the dosage; don't forget to take them (that can sometimes throw you off balance), and never take more than prescribed.

The bad

Before you make any decision to take or not to take antidepressants, make sure that you're fully aware of the potential risks that exist with the use of any medication, particularly those as potent as antidepressants.

Critics charge that many popular antidepressants are unsafe, ineffective, or both. Furthermore, they're associated with side effects that may range from merely uncomfortable to highly dangerous, sometimes even lethal. For example, Wellbutrin (bupropion) can trigger seizures in some patients.

The Food and Drug Administration (FDA) has issued a Public Health Advisory on the use of popular antidepressants by children and adults. Some patients, particularly children, experience increased depression and suicidal thoughts after taking antidepressants. Therefore, both adults and children should be closely monitored, especially at the beginning of treatment, or when the doses are either increased or decreased.

The FDA also cautions that both adults and children taking antidepressants can develop side effects, including anxiety, agitation, panic attacks, insomnia, irritability, hostility, impulsivity, akathisia (severe restlessness), hypomania, and mania. The antidepressants in question include Prozac (fluoxetine); Zoloft (sertraline); Paxil (paroxetine); Luvox (fluvoxamine); Celexa (citalopram); Lexapro (escitalopram); Wellbutrin (bupropion); Effexor (venlafaxine); Serzone (nefazodone); and Remeron (mirtazapine).

But wait, that's not all. Another, lesser known side effect is *tardive dyskinesia,* a medication-induced tic disorder. It most often shows up as involuntary movements usually affecting the mouth, lips and tongue. The tics may be quite disfiguring.

Working with a psychiatrist

If you want medical treatment for depression, we recommend seeking out psychiatrists. Currently, some 70 percent of antidepressant prescriptions are written out by general practitioners, but they aren't always as familiar or as up-to-date on antidepressants as they should be. Besides, a reputable psychiatrist monitors her patients closely for any warning symptoms and is more likely to spot those warnings accurately than doctors who are more familiar with physical ailments.

So you think you're in a rat race . . .

In a study published by the American Psychological Association, Rod K. Dishman, MD, of the University of Georgia used rats to compare exercise to the antidepressant drug imipramine. First, he induced a depression-like condition in these rats by using the drug clomipramine. Then he gave one group of rats 24-hour access to a running-wheel for 12 weeks. Another group ran on a treadmill for an hour a day, six days a week, for 12 weeks. A third group received imipramine for the last six days of the experiment, and a fourth group received no treatment or exercise.

Dr. Dishman determined whether the rats experienced an improvement in depression by detecting an increase in brain concentration of norepinephrine and serotonin metabolism, and an increase in sexual activity. The rats given imipramine and both exercise groups showed the telltale changes in the balance of neurotransmitters. But only the wheel-running rats showed both an improvement in their mood and an increase in sexual activity.

The moral? Exercise is good; exercise that's not forced is even better. (How's your sex life, by the way?)

Even if you don't see a psychiatrist, if you suffer from depression, seek help! Depression, with or without hypoglycemia, is an illness, not a moral weakness. There's absolutely no reason for anyone today to suffer from the debilitating illness of depression without seeking help.

Chapter 11

Making It through Your Day at Work

*H*aving a metabolic disorder such as hypoglycemia doesn't have to unduly complicate your life. With just a few adjustments and modifications, you can circumvent any potential problems that hypoglycemia may pose in your work life. Taking control over hypoglycemia is all about planning and management.

Make your health a priority. You may think that putting your work first is virtuous and will help you get ahead, but in the long run, you're only sabotaging yourself with health problems.

To better manage your health, you may need to let co-workers know about your health challenges. (This doesn't mean coming across as a hypochondriac or someone who's using health issues as an excuse to get special treatment.) This chapter shows you how to inform others of your health concerns in a professional, respectful manner that doesn't undermine your credibility.

We also address the issue of work stress in this chapter. No matter what type of work you do, you're bound to be confronted with stressors, making it that much more difficult to deal with your hypoglycemic symptoms. By taking proactive steps to deal with workday stress, you can ease the symptoms and smooth out potential problems. (For hints on dealing with other stress, flip to Chapter 9.)

No Rings around Either: Blue and White Collar Workers

Because so many different jobs are out there, we can't cover every angle of dealing with hypoglycemia at work. (For work-related legal matters, see "Flying with the legal eagles," later in this chapter.) Whatever your field, whatever your collar color, all jobs offer different challenges, so we can offer only generalities. Only you know the special circumstances and the particulars of your job. It shouldn't be that difficult to accommodate your needs, no matter where you work.

Bad work habits don't just include surfing the Internet

Do you catch yourself working so hard that when you look at the clock you realize that you missed lunch? You may be committed to your job, but when you have hypoglycemia, you need to make sure you take time for yourself at work.

Here are some things that will stress you out; unbalance you physically, mentally, and emotionally; and ultimately lead to problems with blood sugar regulation:

✔ Skipping breakfast

✔ Skipping lunch (If you miss breakfast and/or lunch, you won't be able to work efficiently.)

✔ Shoveling food into your mouth

✔ Not taking enough breaks

✔ Continuing to work when exhausted

✔ Staying up late to finish the day's work

✔ Being a perfectionist

✔ Making negative comments to yourself, like "No one appreciates the work I do."

✔ Failing to communicate with colleagues

✔ Not trusting others to do their share of the work

✔ Needing to validate your self-worth through work

✔ Not asking for help when you need it

✔ Refusing to acknowledge that hypoglycemia is a problem that needs to be treated

To discover how to better manage yourself, turn to Chapters 9 and 16.

Hard hat area

If you engage in physical labor, you have to be especially careful about your blood sugar level. Symptoms such as tremors of the hand, dizziness, and weakness can jeopardize your safety.

Other general rules for hard hat workers include the following:

- ✔ **Eat something every two hours.** This schedule helps you maintain a constant blood sugar level.

- ✔ **Get enough calories.** Your body needs enough calories to function properly. If you're on a weight-reduction diet, you can decrease your calorie intake a bit, but don't overdo it. Eating frequently helps stave off hunger and makes it easier to lose weight.

- ✔ **Consider adding more carbohydrates to your diet.** Depending on how vigorous your work is, you may want to eat a lot more carbs. Consuming roughly 40 percent of your calories in carbohydrates is normally recommended for hypoglycemics. But if you engage in a great deal of physical labor, you can consume up to 60 percent of your calories in carbs. (Chapter 6 tells you more about percentages and portions.)

  Start with a small increase in the amount of carbs you eat, and then gradually increase the amount to see how it makes you feel. If the increase triggers more hypoglycemic symptoms and carbohydrate cravings, cut back.

- ✔ **Eat only high-quality carbs, such as non-starchy veggies, fruits, and whole grains.** If you're one of the many hypoglycemics who can't handle whole grains, eliminate them from your diet regardless of how many calories you burn.

- ✔ **Limit bread to one slice a day, and eat more grains, such as millet and quinoa.** See Chapter 6 for info about healthy foods.

- ✔ **Carry snacks with you wherever you go.** Never, ever go anywhere without food.

Tie required

If you work regular hours in an office, you should be able to eat every two to two-and-a-half hours during breaks and lunch. If your break times aren't regular, and you often forget to take them because you're concentrating on your work, it may be a good idea to

- ✔ Set a wristwatch with multiple alarms.

✔ Have a family member or an answering service call you at pre-arranged times.

✔ Make signs for your desk to remind you to eat.

Addressing Your Boss and Co-Workers

Where are you in terms of work? Are you barely holding your own? Is your work record so spotty that you may be fired? Do you have excessive absenteeism due to your health condition? Or, are you in pretty good shape, just needing a little bit of help from your colleagues to function better?

Depending on your job and your relationship with your superiors, you may be hesitant to approach them with what appears to be a personal problem. You may be especially concerned if your company's corporate culture is cutthroat, and any shortcomings on your part, real or imagined, can be used as ammunition against you. On the other hand, if your health is impacting your work performance, it's not just your problem. You need to work out a solution.

No need to worry though. This section can help you talk to your boss and co-workers. However, depending on your own circumstances, you may be better off not telling your boss the whole story. This section shows you how to walk that fine line.

Knowing when (and how) to tell your boss and co-workers

If your hypoglycemia is affecting your work and work relationships, you may have already considered telling your boss and co-workers why you're taking extra time off or why you're struggling to stay focused in the afternoon.

You may want to discuss matters with Human Resources (HR) before approaching your boss, because HR usually has to clear any special arrangements. Of course, if you have a wonderful rapport with your boss, you may want to go to her first; it helps to have someone on your side.

How do you know whether now is the best time? Discuss the matter if you

- Work somewhere with a policy against eating at your desk, and you can't get away to a breakroom for a snack
- Need extra breaks
- Frequently travel for your job
- Are expected to put in long hours
- Often call in sick
- Have been unable to concentrate, and your performance has suffered

Remember that you have certain rights, and if your health is a matter that needs to be discussed, by all means, do so. You may have more credibility if you get a diagnosis from a medical doctor or other healthcare practitioner before coming out as a hypoglycemic.

Knowing when not to tell

If your condition isn't very severe, and it hasn't impacted your work, then perhaps you don't need to mention it to your supervisor. Consider all your options and your particular situation. You know where you are in the corporate hierarchy (assuming that you work for a corporation) and what your corporate culture is like. If it's a nice, cozy, family-like atmosphere, you may have little to worry about, although there are fewer work places like that today.

If you don't feel comfortable or if your hypoglycemia isn't impacting your job performance, you don't need to disclose anything to your boss or co-workers. However, if your place of employment has sticky rules about, for example, eating at your desk or work space, you may be able to gently ask your supervisor for special permission because of a health issue if you need to eat more often.

Even if you decide not to tell your boss or co-workers about your condition, find at least one ally at work who is caring, trustworthy, and dependable. Perhaps you can ask this person to help you during times when your symptoms flare and you need some extra help coping. When you're in pain or suffering from brain fog and can't trust yourself to eat regularly, you may ask this person to help you remember to eat at predetermined intervals until your condition improves. As an adult, asking someone to remind you to eat may seem weird. You're not in kindergarten, after all! But the point is that when your brain isn't getting its fuel, your thinking function starts to shut down. When your thinking shuts down, you probably aren't going to remember when you have to eat. Explain the physical condition that you have; emphasize that it won't be a permanent arrangement. When your condition stabilizes, you'll be in good enough shape that you won't need these constant reminders.

Flying with the legal eagles

If you decide to tell your supervisor that you're hypoglycemic, first consider becoming familiar with your rights as an employee, especially as they pertain to your health. The Americans with Disabilities Act (ADA) protects your rights as an employee if you're "a qualified individual with disabilities." Who falls under this category? Anyone with a physical or mental impairment that substantially limits one or more major life activities, such as seeing, hearing, speaking, walking, breathing, performing manual tasks, learning, caring for oneself, and working. These disabilities include such conditions as epilepsy, paralysis, HIV infection, and diabetes. Sprains, broken limbs, or the flu won't cut it.

In other words, even if you tell your employer that you have hypoglycemia or a related condition, he can't fire you on the basis of that alone. You have the right to ask your employer for any reasonable accommodations you need to perform the duties assigned to you. Of course, what's reasonable is open to interpretation, but if both parties are acting in good faith, you should be able to work out an arrangement that's satisfactory for everyone concerned.

To protect yourself, follow these steps:

1. **Get a letter or memo, preferably from a medical doctor, explaining your illness.**

   If you can't get the note from a doctor, get it from another health practitioner. Ask for a written diagnosis and medical recommendations. At the very least, try to obtain a written description of your condition for your employer's benefit. Go to someone who's familiar with your symptoms and can confirm the dates you suffered and the specific symptoms.

2. **Ask to speak to your supervisor about your condition privately.**

   If the situation warrants it, you may want to wait until the end of the workday to discuss the matter. Be forthright about your physical condition, because your supervisor needs to be aware of your symptoms.

3. **Keep a written record of any communication between yourself and management, including the date(s) of your meeting with your supervisor and what you talked about.**

You may need to prove that you did your best to work things out, so creating a paper trail is important. Don't announce that you're keeping a file, however. If the meeting with your supervisor doesn't go well, don't discuss it with anyone else in the office, because people may think that you're complaining about management. You don't want to appear to be antagonistic.

If things get out of hand to the point that you receive disciplinary action, you can ask to see what's in your file. Finding out the content of your file is important so that you can figure out what to do. If the information is accurate, try to correct any work problems that have been pointed out. If the information is inaccurate, find a way to correct it. Check with your union steward (if you have one) to see how you can do this. If you aren't in a union, bring up the matter with your direct supervisor, HR rep, or whoever handles such matters.

Finding practical solutions

Before you approach your boss, make a list of the topics you want to discuss and the specific requests you're making. Prepare alternatives for whatever requests you're making.

Bring the supervisor into the process of finding solutions. Be open to her suggestions, but don't put the onus on her to come up with ideas. Make it clear that you're on the same side, trying to find ways to help you be as productive as possible at work.

Some practical solutions to help you cope with hypoglycemia at work include the following:

- ✔ **Offer general information about hypoglycemia's symptoms and how you can prevent them.** An understanding of the condition and the possible need for regular work schedules and meal breaks is usually helpful and appreciated.

- ✔ **Keep a progress report for yourself.** That way, if necessary, you can point out that you're following through on your commitment to work things out responsibly.

- ✔ **Talk privately to co-workers who you may have offended with your mood swings or temper outbursts.** Offer them a sincere apology and tell them what low blood sugar can do to one's brain. It may take a little time, but after you show that you're getting more stable, they may be ready to trust you.

✔ **Eat a small snack before meetings so that you don't have a sudden blood sugar dip.** Even with such precautions, people with a blood sugar imbalance may feel fine one minute and then, suddenly, without warning, feel faint or weak the next. If you're prone to such attacks, bring something to drink with you, such as milk or unsweetened soy milk. These drinks should be enough to forestall a hypoglycemic incident. If you still have problems, ask your supervisor whether you can leave briefly to get a snack.

Framing your condition positively

If you decide the best course of action is to tell your boss and you're ready to talk to him, make sure you plan the discussion and exactly what you're going to say. Come prepared with documentation from your medical provider.

When speaking to your supervisor or management about your condition, follow these simple guidelines:

✔ **Be honest.** Simply state that hypoglycemia is a condition that's related to diabetes, and that you've been advised that it may progress into diabetes if you don't treat it properly. Therefore, you're acting in a responsible manner by taking whatever measures are necessary to prevent your condition from becoming more of a problem.

One caveat: Don't feel compelled to give a blow-by-blow account of every pain and ache you have. Keep the discussion brief and to the point.

✔ **Apologize immediately for any problems or inconveniences that your symptoms may have caused.** Your tone should be one of taking responsibility, not of self-pity or complaint. You don't want to make yourself sound like a hopeless invalid.

✔ **Accept input about where you may have fallen short in your work performance as a result of your physical condition.** If your boss gives no such input, simply point out things you'll do to make sure that your work improves.

✔ **Don't dwell on the problem.** Whatever your challenges, ruminating on them will only make you feel worse. You're more likely to come up with creative solutions if you take a break from thinking about your problem.

✔ **Focus on the positives, not the negatives.** Because you have become more knowledgeable about your condition and are participating in a healthy lifestyle, you can be even more productive than other employees. To effectively live with hypoglycemia, you have to be self-disciplined, self-aware, and self-responsible — all of which are invaluable characteristics that companies look for in their employees.

✔ **Emphasize that you know what the problem is and you're getting a handle on it.** When you learn to control the problem, your condition will stabilize, and you'll fulfill the essential tasks of your employment position.

If you frame requests in a positive way, you're more likely to be heard. At the least, a positive attitude can keep any discussions from turning ugly. Keep in mind that your employer hired you to carry out a specific job; you have an obligation and responsibility to fulfill your duties to the best of your ability.

Putting Up a Cot in the Cubicle? Managing Long Work Hours

Do you work more than 40 hours a week? Surveys show that a rising number of people in the United States are clocking in a record number of hours at work. It's not uncommon for people to put in 18 to 20 hours a day. In fact, Americans are putting in longer hours than most other nations, surpassing even workaholic Japan! We're talking about averages here, of course. Your country of residence doesn't preclude you from working inordinately long hours. It all depends on individual circumstances.

This section helps you understand a bit better your working style and rhythm as well as gives you some ways to break up your workday so you aren't slaving away without any reprieve.

Gettin' in the groove with work

If you want to work efficiently, figure out your personal rhythm and try to work in accordance with it. Different occupations have different rhythms, tempos, and paces. If your natural rhythm isn't in accordance with your job's rhythm, you'll likely wear yourself out.

Ask yourself the following questions:

✔ Am I a morning person or a night owl? (Hypoglycemics tend to do better at night, although there are exceptions.)

✔ Do I work better or worse under deadline pressure?

✔ Do I work in spurts or at an even, constant pace?

Now, ask the following questions in relation to your work:

- ✔ Am I a team player or a lone wolf?
- ✔ Which tasks do I enjoy the most?
- ✔ Which tasks give me the most problems?

By understanding your personal style, you'll be better able to adapt to your working environment. You'll not only feel healthier, but you'll also be able to work more effectively as well. Coping with hypoglycemia means making lifestyle changes, which in turn requires you to do a little soul searching.

Breaking up your work day

Do you work five hours straight without getting up to use the restroom or to snack on healthy food? Are you dragging and have no energy when you need to complete the most important report of the day? If so, taking small, frequent breaks gives you a chance to re-fuel by eating a small snack. Doing so will increase your energy and improve your concentration.

Consider tackling the most troublesome portion of your job when you're the most energetic, and reward yourself with the tasks that you truly enjoy. If you don't like anything about your work, make plans to get into a different line of work. Even if you have to work toward a distant goal, taking concrete action should make your current circumstances easier.

You may want to incorporate the following schedule into your workday:

- ✔ **Take a mini-break every 45 to 60 minutes.** (This is in addition to the official 10 to 15 minute breaks you may get.)

  - Do a few neck rolls and eye rolls, and let your eyes rest by looking out into the distance.

  - Make sure that you blink frequently if you work on a computer for most of the day. (The person who blinks first is *not* the loser.)

  - Do a few *isometrics* (exercises in which you contract certain muscles). For instance, tighten your thigh muscles for a few seconds and then release.

  - Stretch out a little every once in a while. Go to the water cooler or the bathroom.

Don't worry, you're not wasting time. These mini-breaks take just a few minutes, and they make a big difference in your performance and the way you feel. Your focus, concentration, and thinking will be much sharper.

You may, at times, feel more lethargic or cloudy headed than usual. Or you may notice an increase in the intensity of some of your other symptoms. To help alleviate your symptoms, try to schedule your main breaks so that you can physically lie down for 15 minutes (or for a half an hour during lunch). Lying down is much more restorative than sitting. If lying down just isn't possible, perhaps you can put your head down on your desk and close your eyes. Even resting with your head down on your desk can make a world of difference.

✓ **Eat every 1½ to 2 hours.** This tip is especially important for maintaining your blood sugar. You won't lose any time. We're not talking a banquet here. You can snack while you're working. Try nibbling on nuts or seeds. Or bring plain yogurt or cottage cheese.

✓ **Eat more protein for lunch.** When you start your hypoglycemic diet, you may begin to notice that you don't have post-lunch drowsiness and mid-afternoon slumps like you used to. If you still have problems, cut back drastically on starches such as pasta and grains.

Preparing for those long hours when you're away from the office

On your days off or after a day on the job, take a moment for yourself. Take care of your physical and emotional self in the following ways:

✓ **At the end of the day or on days off, allow yourself to rest without guilt.**

- Get other members of the family to do household chores, such as cleaning or the laundry. Or hire help.

- Eat out instead of cooking at home (if you think it will help). Just make sure that you order something within your diet plan, such as salad, steamed vegetables, and grilled fish or chicken.

✓ **Work out at least three times a week but don't overdo it.** Don't become a weekend warrior who crams in hours of exercise on days off. (Check out Chapter 8 for more on incorporating exercise into your daily routine.)

✔ **Ask yourself whether you really need to work all those hours.** Keep a written record of all your activities during the day. When you review the account, you'll be able to see where the time wasters are, what can be eliminated or reduced, and where you can improve efficiency. The idea is to work smarter, not harder.

Diffusing Work-Related Stress

Work has stresses all its own — stresses different from those in your personal life. Isn't that nice? Here's how you can deal with these special stresses:

 ✔ **It may sound trite, but live one day at a time.** When something goes wrong at work, remind yourself that this too shall pass. Will anyone care about it 100 years from now? Will *you* care about it in a year?

 ✔ **Eliminate the stressors that can be avoided, and learn to handle everyday stress through meditation and exercise.** (See Chapter 9 for info on how to reduce stress.) Remember that managing stress is a big part of attaining and maintaining health.

 ✔ **Go away for a mini-retreat if you can.** Take an entire weekend off where you aren't interrupted and have time to relax, pamper yourself, and perhaps review your work and career goals. Where are you in your career right now? Where do you want to be? Should you quit your current job? Play for a promotion? Go into a different line of work? Go back to school? Write your memoir? Become a mime?

 ✔ **Have fun.** This agenda item may not be on your radar screen when you're overworked, but scheduling some fun time into every day is important, even if it's for only 10 minutes. Have lunch with someone you enjoy. Go window shopping. Read the funnies. Sketch a drawing. Call a friend and shoot the breeze. At least once a week, try to do something pleasurable that takes a couple of hours or more. For extra enjoyment and relaxation, get a weekly massage if you can afford it. If not, trade massages with family or friends. It's all about inner and outer balance.

The following sections provide plenty of helpful pointers to survive work-related stress. First and foremost, we assist you in looking inward at how your job really affects your life and health. We also give you some ways to help you cope with a stressful job, including staying away from caffeine and making your home away from home a little cozier.

The 6:00 unwind

Unwinding after working a stressful day is hard. Be careful, because overwork can cause your adrenals to become overactive and hypervigilant, thus triggering panic attacks. To relax, instead of reaching for a stiff drink — which is taboo for hypoglycemics — try doing one of the following:

✔ Practice deep breathing.

✔ Meditate.

✔ Participate in a yoga class.

✔ Take a long, relaxing bath with epsom salts.

✔ Listen to some music and read a good book. It has been discovered that watching TV or getting on the computer at night can interfere with sound sleep.

✔ Sleep well. When you're working more than normal, you need to get as deep and restful a sleep as possible. In order to get restorative sleep at night, sleep in a dark room or wear eye shades. Remove all electrical appliances with flashing lights from your bedroom; these appliances have been shown to impede deep sleep.

Evaluating your life: Does this job impede your health?

If your work is seriously detracting from your quality of life and contributing to your poor health, take this opportunity to do a major life review. If you're in poor health, or if you're having a constellation of symptoms (maybe even a galaxy of them), something's not right, whether it's physical, mental, emotional, or spiritual. Your body's metabolic imbalance may be a reflection of an imbalance in your life. To become completely well, you're going to have to address your health in a multi-faceted way, physically, mentally, emotionally, and spiritually. Work occupies most of your waking time; how healthy can you become if your job is a source of major dissatisfaction? The stress of doing work you're not suited for can only exacerbate your hypoglycemia.

Postpone making any major decisions until you have your diet under control and your symptoms have abated. Making sound decisions is hard when your thinking is fuzzy and you're not functioning very well. You can get at least some of your symptoms under control through herbs and supplements. (For a list of herbs and supplements, refer to Chapter 7.) If your main problem is anxiety and depression, and natural remedies aren't helping, try medication. (To read about anxiety and depression, and medicine's role in treating these conditions, turn to Chapter 10.)

Of course, only you can decide what the best course of action is. If you love your job, or if you desperately need the income, sit down and figure out exactly how you need to change your work arrangement. If a reasonable effort to change things on your part meets with no results, you and your job may have to part ways. Make sure that you get yourself a parachute before you take that leap, though! Not having a job can be very stressful.

Passing up the caffeine

Java. The bean. Joe. Whatever you call it, it seems that everybody is drinking coffee in the morning. Many people can't even function without caffeine as an eye-opener. But in fact, too much caffeine actually adds to stress by making your body more prone to releasing *adrenaline*, the stress hormone. Caffeine can also trigger hypoglycemic symptoms, which definitely add to any work stress you may already experience.

Caffeine is detrimental to hypoglycemics. If you're addicted to coffee (you get a headache when you've gone awhile without a mug, even if you drink only a cup a day), taper your use gradually. If you try to stop cold turkey, you'll get a headache. Although not exactly like coffee, substitutes can provide you with the pleasure and comfort of a nice, hot beverage. Try out different substitutes to find the one you enjoy the most. The following list provides some good ways to help you make the transition from coffee to some healthy alternatives:

- ✔ **Find good caffeine-free coffee substitutes.** These may include grain coffees or herbal teas. Decaffeinated coffee is also a no-no because it still contains some caffeine.

- ✔ **Drink green tea or herbal tea.** You may want to try Japanese barley tea (mugi-cha), which doesn't have caffeine.

- ✔ **Make a protein smoothie with protein powder, or create your own favorite drink.** Having protein helps stabilize your blood sugar. Avoid using sugar or artificial sweeteners in your drink.

- ✔ **Mix up some hot chocolate with carob powder and nut or rice milk, and add some stevia to sweeten.** *Carob,* a natural chocolate substitute, doesn't contain stimulants. It also helps normalize hypoglycemia.

✔ **Drink the following morning elixir.** If you really feel that you can't get going in the morning without that little zing of java, try this morning elixir from *IBS For Dummies,* by Carolyn Dean, MD, ND, and L. Christine Wheeler, MA (Wiley). Combine a quart of water, the juice of one lemon, a pinch of cayenne, and the contents of one capsule of ginger.

The ginger helps subdue any possible nausea that you may feel from changing your diet, and the cayenne gets your circulation going and keeps your hands and feet warm — a real boon for hypoglycemics who tend to get cold hands and feet. Some recipes for this drink use about ⅛ teaspoon of cayenne, but to start, use just a pinch of this powerful healer. If you find this drink too sour, add ⅛ teaspoon of stevia, if you're able to tolerate it.

If you absolutely must drink some coffee

✔ **Don't drink coffee on an empty stomach.** It can be very hard on your stomach; besides, it really wreaks havoc on your blood sugar.

✔ **Drink coffee with lots of cream or whole milk.** The protein and fat in the cream will help stabilize your blood sugar (somewhat) and mitigate the negative effects of the caffeine. (Remember, cream does add calories, and it's not for you if you're allergic or lactose intolerant.)

✔ **Take extra B-complex tabs.** Coffee is believed to deplete the vitamin B in your system.

✔ **Cut way back.** If you just can't resist tasting coffee, take a few sips and leave the rest.

Need a quick pick-me-up? Take deep, decaffeinated breaths. You can go to the bathroom or the lounge and meditate for a few minutes, too. Or, if you have an official break time or lunch, walk around the building. If you have enough time, you may even decide to go to the gym. But don't skip your lunch to do so.

Creating a cozy cubicle

Cubicles are just as much a part of some working cultures as coffee drinking. Most people spend the majority of their waking time at work, so you should create as healthy and as pleasant an environment as you can.

To lessen a stressful work environment, you can make your cubicle or work office a little cozier and a lot less stressful with the following ideas:

✔ **Reduce the noise.** Noise pollution can add to stress, which in turn can exacerbate hypoglycemic symptoms. If the noise in your work environment bothers you, get a *white noise generator*. These machines can deflect unwanted sounds and mask discordant noise by producing a smooth sound of rushing air that creates a sense of calm. Some of them even produce a variety of low frequency digital sounds, including the sounds of a lakeshore, rain, surf, a brook, and a waterfall.

✔ **Use environmentally sound cleaning products.** People whose bodies are very sensitive, like most low blood sugar sufferers, are better off using only environmentally sound cleaning products at home and in the office. Some particularly susceptible people may become acutely ill if they work in offices that suffer from *sick building syndrome* (buildings with a high degree of indoor pollution). This often occurs in insulated buildings with windows that don't open. You may not clean your own office, but if you discover anything at work that you're allergic to, find out how you can avoid exposure.

✔ **Get an air purifier.** If the quality of the air in your workplace is a problem, an air purifier can help. Keeping plants on your desk can also help; if nothing else, they can enliven your work space.

✔ **Play some soft music.** Music can have the same calming effect as tranquilizers. Play relaxing music while you work. Just make sure that you don't bother your co-workers.

✔ **Keep healthy snacks close by.** Do you have a co-worker who always sets out a bowl of candies for everyone? To avoid temptation, don't even get close to it. If you have some healthy snacks nearby, chances are you won't be as tempted.

✔ **Ask your company to stock healthy snacks in vending machines.** Office vending machines are bad news. You'll make it easier for yourself if you make them off limits. If you can think of a healthy food item you want that can be sold through a vending machine, ask the vending company to carry it. Call the company directly, or waylay the guy who stocks the machines.

✔ **Ask co-workers to bring in healthier snacks.** Do they wheel danishes and donuts into your office every morning? If so, find out whether they can also start bringing in healthier treats so that people have a choice. Because so many people are on weight-reducing diets these days, you may find a lot of supporters.

Part IV

Spinning a Network of Support for Yourself (and Others)

In this part . . .

Whoever said that no man is an island unto himself was certainly right. Everyone needs the support of other people from time to time; nobody can make it completely alone. In this part, we show you how to set up a support network so that you don't fall on your face while you're dealing with the side effects and aftereffects of hypoglycemia. After all, everyone is bound to suffer at times from low moods and self-doubts. When you're feeling down, you can open the book to this section and discover how to get through those trying times.

This part also addresses those people closest to you. They may not completely understand this condition, so Chapter 14 gives them the support they need to better figure out how hypoglycemia affects you the way it does.

Chapter 12

Jockeying for Support

Supportive people in your life can help you live longer. Or maybe they just make you feel like you live longer; either way, it works. The fact is, humans are naturally social creatures — homo sapiens would never have survived without banding together in groups. In many, many ways, everyone is dependent on everyone else. (Yes, even you, Mr. Macho Man.)

You need the support of others to help you deal with your hypoglycemia. Without it, you may end up wallowing when you could be much happier. This chapter helps you garner that support from, most importantly, yourself, support groups, and a buddy. (Check out Chapter 13 for info on getting support from your friends and family.)

Grasping the Link between Support and Hypoglycemia

Now this little exercise isn't the least bit scientific (so don't quote us or shoot us), but think about what low blood sugar could mean metaphorically: Sugar and sweets often symbolize love. So perhaps you can link low blood sugar to lack of love (if you're in love, and your partner has hypoglycemia, check out Chapter 14), or at least to the perception that you're not getting the tender loving care that you need. Perhaps you're surrounded by loving people, but you've walled yourself off from their love. Maybe you need to mend some rifts in your relationships, or maybe you need to establish new relationships. Aside from the physiological basis for addictions, a craving for sugar can mean a craving for love. (By the way, we're not suggesting that a high blood sugar level means that you're getting too much love — it means that you have sugar in

your blood, but your cells aren't getting their share. So with both
conditions, you're being effectively starved of fuel.)

Whatever your situation, you need to review your health and relationship history if you want to get your blood sugar under control.
A growing body of social and scientific evidence points to the vital
importance of social contact in the maintenance of your health.

You can start by first reviewing your health history. (Chapter 3
shows you how to observe your symptoms.) Then jot down the
names of all the people with whom you have important relationships. This list should include family members, lovers, friends,
teachers, and social contacts who are significant to you. No need
to write long essays (unless you enjoy that); a few well-chosen
words will do. Write down how you feel about these people and
your interactions with them. If you're feeling ambitious, see
whether you notice any connection between the foods you eat and
the people you hang out with. Maybe your mother loves to eat, and
she always entices you to eat forbidden foods. Or maybe your ex-
boyfriend loved to tempt you with chocolates.

Getting Yourself Out There

You can't get support from your friends and family if you don't ask
for it. And to ask for it, you have to make yourself accessible and
available to the people who matter most.

You're thinking, but what if I live alone? What if I work 12-hour days
and am too pooped to go out? What if everyone dearest to me lives
in another state or even another country?

You can't expect your family and friends to read your mind. (Check
out Chapter 13 for more on how you can ask your friends and family
to actually help.) You have to reach out to them and call them regularly. Make yourself — and your phone company — happy. If you're
cost-conscious, there are great long-distance deals available, as well
as cheap, pre-paid phone cards. And if you're set up with broad-
band, you can call for free via the Internet. Explore your options.

If you don't have a family — even a far-flung one — and you don't
have a social network, take immediate action to start getting connected to people. Start by getting involved with

  ✔ Community organizations (such as the YMCA)

  ✔ Social groups sponsored by your particular house of worship

  ✔ Classes that interest you (as opposed to those that don't
    interest you)

- ✔ Workshops and seminars

- ✔ Volunteer activities

- ✔ Professional or trade associations

- ✔ Support groups for hypoglycemics (more on this later in this chapter)

- ✔ Health or fitness groups

You can find information about these types of groups in your local newspaper or on the Internet.

 Get a pet if you can, especially if you live alone and feel isolated. You can get a cat, dog, rabbit, lizard, parakeet, finch, goldfish, or whatever . . . anything that you can love and enjoy taking care of. Studies show that owning and caring for a pet can not only relieve isolation but also reduce family arguments and lead to lower levels of anxiety and depression and fewer illnesses.

 You may be wondering how any of this relates to low blood sugar. It does! Because to properly treat yourself, you need to look at every aspect of your life. Hypoglycemia is often called a *lifestyle illness*. Its treatment depends more on your diet and lifestyle than on medication or any medical, surgical, or high-tech interventions.

Getting to Know Me

First things first. Get your food program in order (see Chapter 6). Then write down exactly how you want to feel, and figure out ways to rearrange your life to best support your journey back to health. (Chapter 16 offers ideas to get you started.) For this purpose, sit down and have a get-acquainted-with-yourself session. You can have this session alone or with someone you trust.

Don't pull the trigger

When it comes to hypoglycemia, what most often derails a treatment program? Food! Food is the biggie, all right. So sit down and brainstorm on all the triggers that can fire your craving for forbidden foods. Write down every single trigger — things, people, or situations that can set off bad eating — that you can think of.

Triggers can be social situations, going to restaurants, losing your pet goldfish, winning the lottery, and so on. Under each trigger, write down what you can do to avoid getting derailed. Go on, wow everyone's socks off with your creative solutions. (For tips and ideas, see Chapter 16.)

If you decide to have a get-acquainted-with-yourself session with someone at your side, make sure that you choose someone who's trustworthy and supportive. You don't need negativity, criticism, or put-downs. ("Oh hell, honey, you don't have blood sugar problems, you just need a brain transplant.")

To become better acquainted with yourself, follow these steps:

1. **Get a notebook and write down everything you're going to do to get healthy.**

   Break the list down into the following categories:

   - Physical goals

     - How would you like to look and feel right now?

     - How is your health?

   - Diet

     - Are you keeping a food journal? (See Chapter 6.)

     - Are you keeping track of what foods you should eat and what foods you should avoid? (See Chapter 6 for a list.)

   - Vitamins, supplements, and herbs

     - What vitamins and supplements are you taking? (Check out Chapter 7 for more info.)

     - In what quantity are you taking them?

   - Medication

     - What medications are you taking?

     - In what quantity are you taking them?

     - Are you setting up and keeping appointments with healthcare practitioners and therapists?

   - Exercise plan

     - What are your current measurements (chest, waist, hips, and so on)?

     - What is your current weight?

     - What exercise plan are you going to follow?

     - How many times a week will you exercise?

     - How long will you exercise each time?

   - Meditation, relaxation, and deep breathing

     - How often are you meditating?

     - How long do your sessions last?

2. **Write exactly how the symptoms caused by your low blood sugar have affected you in each of the following areas:**

   - Health (see Chapter 3)
   - Family
   - Relationships
   - Work/career (see Chapter 11)
   - Short- and long-term goals
   - Leisure activities

3. **Write how you can avoid the problems caused by your symptoms.**

   - Health and energy level
     - Exercises (see Chapter 8)
     - Meditation/breathing (see Chapter 9)
     - Herbs, vitamins, and supplements (see Chapter 7)
   - Job (see Chapter 11)
     - How can you manage your symptoms at work?
     - What can you tell your supervisors about your health condition?
   - Managing your moods (Chapter 10)
     - Should you consider antidepressants?
     - How can you deal with anger?

4. **Write what you think life will be like when you're free of major symptoms.**

   - Family
     - How much time are you spending with your family?
     - How can you and your family have more fun together?
   - Relationship goals
     - What would you like your significant relationship to be like?
     - What can you do to achieve your ideal relationship?
   - Support system choice
     - What can you do to develop new friendships?
     - How can you find groups with similar health goals?

- Spiritual needs

  - What are you doing to meet your needs? Religious/spiritual practices? Groups? Literature?

  - How can you deepen your relationship with others who have a similar spiritual bent?

- Career goals

  - How do you feel about your job? Are you satisfied?

  - Where would you like to be? How will you achieve your goal?

- Educational goals

  - Are you in school? Do you want to enroll in school?

  - What would you like to accomplish?

- Others goals or concerns

  - Do you want to start a new hobby?

  - Do you want to improve another area of life that isn't listed here?

 Choose three goals that you want to reach within the next year. Pick something that's easily attainable so that you can get a sense of accomplishment. Every month, review what you've written so that you can see how your objectives or perspectives may have changed. Note whether you're feeling more satisfied with life in general as your health improves.

Joining the In-Crowd

Your family may be the best place to turn for help (check out Chapter 13). However, sometimes your family just can't or doesn't understand, and you need people who truly understand what you're going through. Because humans are social creatures, support groups give you the motivation to stick with a program that's not always easy. Over the long term, members of a group are often much better at accomplishing their goals. Go to local community centers or call hospitals to find groups specific to hypoglycemia.

 Admittedly, groups for hypoglycemia aren't as plentiful as those for other ailments. If you can't find a hypoglycemia-specific group, sign up for groups that have informational or support meetings about health and healing.

Or why not organize your own support group for hypoglycemia? If you get involved with starting a support group, you may find it easier to feel motivated. Okay, get the ball rolling! Don't get bogged down in details. You don't have to wait until you find an ideal meeting place for the group. Start with these steps:

1. **Call up everyone you know who may be interested in joining a support group for hypoglycemia.**

   Ask friends, neighbors, and colleagues whether they're interested in joining your group. You can also ask them whether they know anyone else who may have low blood sugar.

2. **Put up flyers and ads promoting your group.**

   You can post messages on relevant Internet forums, or post them in clinics, hospitals, universities, or churches. (Get permission first.) You can also put them up in your neighborhood supermarket, if there is a community bulletin board.

3. **Start your own Web site or newsletter.**

   For more info, check out *Creating Web Pages For Dummies,* 8th Edition, by Bud E. Smith and Arthur Bebak (Wiley).

4. **Decide on a meeting place.**

   Consider meeting at the homes of members. If that isn't feasible, you can usually meet at libraries and bookstores for free, and they may be more accessible for drop-ins. You may even be able to get a group discount by purchasing books on hypoglycemia or other related subjects at bookstores where you frequently meet.

5. **Consider charging a membership fee.**

   Discuss what you think is a fair amount to charge participants. You want to be able to cover expenses and have some money left over for other purposes, such as inviting speakers or financing creative events. Charging a membership fee for the group may make people value it more. Freebies just can't get respect.

Netting some help

Finding online support groups — those you can contact through the Internet — for hypoglycemics may be easier than finding groups that meet in person. Key phrases to enter into a search engine are **hypoglycemia, support groups,** or **low blood sugar.** You can find numerous online support groups where you can discuss any issues you're working through. (Check out the nearby sidebar "Finding more support on the Web" for specific resources.)

Finding more support on the Web

The World Wide Web offers plenty of support if you feel like you're fighting a never-ending battle against hypoglycemia. Check out the following:

- ✔ **eHealth Forum (http://ehealthforum.com/health/hypoglycemia.html):** An online community with a forum for health and medical questions, including those related to hypoglycemia. Only registered members can post messages, but anyone can read the messages. Membership is free. The site also offers articles on popular health topics.

- ✔ **HELP: Institute for Body Chemistry (http://home.earthlink.net/~ekrimmel2):** This national network was founded in 1979 by Edward and Patricia Krimmel. It provides support and information for people interested in body chemistry, especially as it relates to hypoglycemia. It also promotes research between food and body chemistry, and provides assistance in starting support groups. For information or assistance, send an e-mail to Patricia at ekrimmel2@earthlink.net, or send snail mail to: 6 Mellon Terrace, Pittsburgh, PA 15206.

- ✔ **How Does Hypoglycemia Affect Our Lives? (www.hypoinfo.com):** This site features a comprehensive listing of articles and information about hypoglycemia, real-life stories of hypoglycemics, links to other sites, and a forum for discussions related to hypoglycemia.

- ✔ **Hypoglycemia Forum (http://hypoglycemia.itgo.com):** The Hypoglycemia Forum Web site offers support and information to hypoglycemics and their family members. The site features a message board and several links to other helpful Web sites.

- ✔ **The Hypoglycemia Support Foundation, Inc. (www.hypoglycemia.org):** This foundation was founded in 1980. The Web site provides book, audio, and other products; diet information; surveys; and an online newsletter.

Be careful when you post messages online. We're not talking Big Brother here, but unlike the spoken word, your written words are stored, and the chance exists that someone, somewhere, can use them against you. It's not likely, but a little caution never hurt anyone. Remember, too, that people you meet online can pretend to be anyone they want to be. People can, and do, try on different identities and different genders. Luckily, this practice is much more common in groups devoted to the dating game; most of the people involved in hypoglycemic groups are sincerely engaged in getting their blood sugar levels under control and helping others do the same.

Eat before you type

Spending hours surfing the Internet can be all too easy. Before you go online, make sure that you eat something. You may want to set a timer or alarm clock to remind you to eat your next snack or meal. Keeping your blood sugar regulated is important. You don't want to get irritated and send nasty messages that you later regret. Some otherwise sweet people can undergo a sudden transformation and lash out at nothing in particular when their blood sugar is low. After they eat and restore themselves to sanity, they then spend an inordinate amount of time apologizing to the hapless recipients of their e-mail. If this pattern of behavior sounds familiar, post a reminder note by your computer: Eat before you write. Don't send messages when annoyed.

You may not see anyone's face (unless you have a Web camera), and you may be able to hide behind your computer screen, but that doesn't mean you have a license to be rude. Extend the same courtesy you show when interacting face to face. Don't spread rumors, send unsolicited ads, or insult people. Everyone is entitled to his opinion. And when you're involved with support groups, all your personal information should be kept confidential.

If you spend a great part of your time in front of the computer already, try to participate in real flesh-and-blood groups in addition to, or in lieu of, online support. You can't substitute for face-to-face experience. But chat groups, message boards, and e-mails are convenient ways to contact people. You may also be able to develop a good rapport with people online.

Doing the 12-step

Twelve-step groups help members overcome various addictions by following a series of (surprise!) 12 steps. If you can't find a good hypoglycemic group, and you don't want to start one of your own, 12-stepping may be the solution for you. (If you're looking for a dance group, try classes.)

The following are some advantages to joining a 12-step program:

- ✔ They offer support to those who are desperate, whether that desperation stems from illness, addiction, unhealthy relationship dependencies, or other emotional issues. (Bring plenty of tissues if you tend to get teary-eyed.)

- ✔ You can easily find a meeting in virtually any community. There seem to be more 12-step groups than other types of support groups. If you'd rather talk face to face, physically attending a group is your best bet.

 ✔ You don't have to pay dues or fees. You may make voluntary
    contributions.

You may feel isolated when trying to deal with your low blood sugar
problem. You may feel as though no one else has to face the same
challenges. But when you sit in these meetings, you'll most likely
come away with the realization that everyone has her own cross to
bear. You may also come to realize that when the you-know-what
hits the fan, some people will help you clean it up. You're not alone.
You can go to weekly meetings, and you can collect telephone numbers and personal contacts if you wish. You can also get a one-on-
one sponsor to help you overcome hurdles. The following sections
focus on some 12-step groups you may want to try.

Overeaters Anonymous

If you can't find a group specific to hypoglycemia, Overeaters
Anonymous (OA) may be of value. A general misconception is that
you have to be overweight to join OA. Not so. Meetings are also
available for those suffering with bulimia or anorexia, two eating
disorders.

OA focuses on issues with food; it doesn't necessarily focus on
weight loss or advocate any one type of diet. It addresses physical,
emotional, and spiritual well-being. OA can be a good choice for
hypoglycemics who may have some emotional issues with food. If,
no matter what you do, you can't seem to curb your cravings, OA
may be a good forum for you. You can share with others the difficulty of trying to adhere to a healthy diet.

Alcoholics Anonymous

Alcoholics Anonymous (AA) is for those who want to recover from,
or are in the process of recovering from, alcoholism. Alcoholism
isn't unusual in hypoglycemics, because faulty glucose metabolism
may be at the root of the addiction in the first place. (See Chapter 2
for more on alcoholism and low blood sugar.) If you have parents
who are alcoholics, you're likely to have either drinking problems
or hypoglycemia. Or maybe both.

If your drinking is getting out of hand, you should definitely consider following the basic hypoglycemic diet and either enroll yourself in a treatment program for alcoholics or join AA. Sticking to
your diet may also help you control your alcohol problems.

Emotions Anonymous

Emotions Anonymous (EA) is for people who have difficulty dealing with their emotions. This group can help you deal with the
emotions and mood swings that may be caused, in part, by your
erratic blood sugar.

Avoiding cults

When you're in a physically and psychologically vulnerable state as a result of your hypoglycemia, having some guidelines can help clarify matters. If you manage to estrange everyone around you and are desperate to be admitted to a group — any group — the possible danger rings even more true. And if it's anything like the first time you felt accepted and cared for, you're wide open for manipulation.

So what's a cult? Having a doctrine doesn't make a group of people a cult. Even claiming that drinking your own urine will heal you of hypoglycemia doesn't make a group of people a cult. (That just makes 'em wacky.) Although we have no hard and fast rules for what officially constitutes a cult, watch out for certain signs. The following list provides some warnings you should be on the lookout for. The list isn't comprehensive, and not every cult displays all these characteristics, but if you notice even a few of these signs, consider them a red flag:

- ✔ The group has a pyramid-type, authoritarian leadership structure.

- ✔ They claim to be the only way to truth, happiness, and healing from hypoglycemia or whatever else ails you.

- ✔ They use mind-control techniques on their members that may include subtle brainwashing to make members feel that they're the special "chosen" ones or that the outside world is evil and dangerous.

- ✔ They use intimidation, such as belittling or actual threats of violence, to keep members in line.

- ✔ They discourage or attempt to cut off your relationships with family and friends.

- ✔ They believe that they're right and everyone else is wrong.

- ✔ They pressure you to give all that you can to the group — all your money and possessions, for instance.

If you find yourself involved in a group like this, run, don't walk! Cut off all contact with them. Getting out is easier at the first warning sign than after you've been involved for a long time. Don't succumb to pressure to return. Go to a therapist who's knowledgeable about cults. Enlist the support of your family.

Don't look for medical or psychiatric service from EA groups, and don't expect personal or family counseling. Just like all other 12-step groups, EA groups aren't professionally run organizations, but the famous 12 steps give the groups structure and unity.

EA addresses a wide variety of emotional issues, including depression, anger, broken or strained relationships, grief, anxiety, low self-esteem, panic, abnormal fears, resentment, jealousy, guilt, despair, boredom, loneliness, withdrawal, obsessive and negative thinking, worry, and compulsive behavior. (Chapter 3 talks about the symptoms of hypoglycemia.)

Buddying Up

With the buddy system, you pair up with a friend and help each other attain a goal you both want. For instance, you may both want to change your diet. The buddy system works by making you accountable for what you've agreed to do for your own benefit. Cheating or sliding can be all too easy if you're the only one taking account of your actions. When you have a friend who you have to answer to, meeting your self-imposed goal (which may be to quit eating sugar or start exercising) somehow becomes much more important.

Keep a telephone handy so that you can call your buddy when the following situations arise:

- ✔ You can't stick to your exercise program.
- ✔ You're tempted to go off your diet.
- ✔ You're just having a bad day.
- ✔ You're craving sugar because you're lonely, angry, or depressed.

Listening to your buddy's problems will help you, as well. In fact, you may begin to form a bond. When your buddy has a success, you'll feel as though you have had a success, as well. Your buddy's success may motivate you to reach your own health goals. When you have someone pulling for you, you don't want to let that person down. And when you're responsible for someone else, you're less likely to cheat.

This section helps you locate a suitable buddy and tells you what you can do to start building a satisfying relationship with your buddy.

Matching up with a buddy

Do you want a buddy to help you through the bad times and who you can celebrate the good times? If so, the question is, "How can I find a buddy?" Who should you pair up with?

The best place to start is to pair up with anyone who has a similar goal or concern, and who you can trust to keep up the alliance. Find someone else who's concerned with low blood sugar. If you can't find someone who has hypoglycemia and wants to work on a recovery program, remember that plenty of people want to lose weight. So pair up with someone who's trying to shed some pounds or cut sugar from his diet.

Because your goals will be similar, you'll probably work well together. You'll both need to exercise, and many foods that are off-limits for you are also banned from weight-reduction diets. Differences are sure to occur, so you don't need to follow the same diet. Just explain to each other what you intend to do, and make sure that your partner keeps his word. You need to be caring and compassionate, but strict. Don't let your partner slip up, and vice versa. Be willing to scold each other in a caring, supportive way.

Starting off on the right foot with your buddy

No matter who your buddy is, you want to make sure that you're both on the same page and that you both have the same expectations from each other.

 At the initial meeting between you and your buddy, you need to

✓ **Establish a meeting frequency.**

- Depending on your schedule, agree to meet weekly or biweekly. You'll lose momentum if you go longer between meetings.

- Determine what you want to do during your meetings. Set time aside to meditate together or read quotes from inspirational books.

- Agree on a time when you can call to check up on your progress. Ideally, you should call every day; send an e-mail instead if works better for you. You don't have to have a long-winded conversation — two to five minutes will suffice for a daily check-in. When you're experiencing difficulties that can throw you off track, schedule a longer conversation to discuss them with your buddy.

✓ **Establish your goals.** Be very clear on what you want to accomplish. For example, if your goal is to start keeping a food journal, put that down in writing. Tell your buddy your goal.

✔ **Determine how you'll meet your goals.** You need a plan to get where you want to go. Write out exactly how you'll achieve your goal. Your goal can be as simple as buying a notebook for your food journal and carrying it around with you.

✔ **Share literature so that you can better understand what the other person needs.** Ask your buddy to show you relevant information on whatever he's working on. For example, if his goal is to quit smoking, agree to read any information he may have about smoking and how to quit the habit. Likewise, share any books you have about hypoglycemia. You don't have to read everything; just enough to get an understanding of the issues your buddy is facing.

✔ **Show your buddy everything you write down in terms of your wants and needs.** If you don't write everything down, you'll forget. After you write it down, then share it with your buddy so that you don't have any misunderstandings.

✔ **Explain your diet and the concept.** (See Chapter 6 for diet information.) Your buddy needs to understand the diet you're following and why so he can better support you in your efforts to stick to your diet. He won't be able to support you effectively if he doesn't understand how important your diet is to your recovery.

✔ **Discuss rewards.** When you meet your goals, take turns rewarding each other. You can give each other a massage, go to a movie or for a hike, or do anything that you find pleasurable. (Don't use food as a reward!) This is one sweet alliance that won't cause your blood sugar to come crashing down.

The downside of the buddy system is the possibility that one or both of you may slip up on your commitments to yourselves and to each other. You can falter despite the best of intentions. Maybe your hypoglycemic symptoms are too much for you to handle; or you have other things going on that demand more of your time; or you find that you're paired up with the wrong person. If you slip up, don't despair. Discuss it with your buddy to see whether you both want to give the buddy system another shot, change what you're doing, or just drop it. If you decide that the partnership isn't working out, you may want to find someone else.

Chapter 13

Dealing with Family and Friends: Eat and Let Eat

. . . .

In This Chapter

▶ Talking to your loved ones about hypoglycemia

▶ Communicating your needs

▶ Sticking to your diet in the face of naysayers

. . . .

*T*he world would be fine and splendid if you could always count on those nearest and dearest to you to be your most enthusiastic cheerleaders. They're the ones who exert the most power over you. Yet the sad truth is that, instead of inspiring you, your friends and family often are the very ones who drag you down. They may well be good, decent people who have the most honorable intentions, but they can still thwart your attempt to regain your health.

Your first task, therefore, is to help your loved ones understand this admittedly perplexing syndrome. After they understand it, they may be much more willing to support your recovery process. Then and only then can you proceed to ask them for help in changing your lifestyle and dealing with the symptoms of hypoglycemia. Don't assume that they'll automatically know what to do; you have to let them know exactly what you need from them. Present your requests clearly and directly, and don't place blame on anyone.

This chapter gives you the tools to communicate your wants effectively — specifically in terms of changing your diet — and shows you how to deal with your family and friends.

How Hypoglycemia Can Affect Your Relationships

When it comes to hypoglycemia, most people, perhaps even those individuals closest to you, may not be very sympathetic or helpful.

Why is this? Well, first of all, regardless of how wretched it may make you feel, hypoglycemia is generally not life threatening. Secondly, people still tend to believe that it's all in your head or that you're just malingering. Perhaps in their opinion you were doing just fine before, so why this sudden and drastic attempt to change?

The emotional repercussions of hypoglycemia can take a toll on relationships. If you suffer from blood sugar imbalance, your brain isn't getting enough glucose, its primary fuel. It's like sputtering along in a car with an almost-empty tank. You're not operating at your best, and you're not feeling your best. Studies have shown that when a person is suffering from hypoglycemia, judgment becomes clouded, and the person becomes easily irritable, even irrational. Add to that depression and constant mood swings — and you can see how difficult it can be for family and friends to deal with a hypoglycemic (check out Chapter 14, which speaks directly to your loved ones).

Explaining to Your Significant Other

People who have normal metabolism sometimes can't understand the energy fluctuations your low blood sugar causes. These fluctuations are one of the first things you need to help your loved ones understand, and this section can help.

Starting with open dialog

You probably don't need to be reminded that absolute and complete honesty is critical in any relationship. And when you're talking about something as important as your health, you owe it to your partner to come completely clean. Even if you're afraid of being judged, if you don't discuss your health issue openly, you'll never win your partner over to your side or at least help him gain some understanding of what living with a metabolic syndrome like hypoglycemia means.

To start off, try to make your conversation as simple as possible. Don't overwhelm your partner with a lot of unimportant or irrelevant information. Get to the point, be focused, and stay positive.

To convey information about your condition, take a cue from the politicians:

- ✔ **Prepare your statements in advance so that you don't become confused and forget the important points.** Write out exactly what you're going to say and memorize it. Don't simply blurt out an explanation, or you may say the wrong things.

- ✔ **Collect and present literature about hypoglycemia.** People tend to believe what's in print. Gathering info shows that you've done some homework and aren't just giving a vapid excuse as to why you've been encountering health challenges.

- ✔ **Try not to look like you're announcing a stock market crash.** A talk doesn't need to be deadly serious. You can be informal but informative. Or, conversely, you can ham it up — go all out and type out written statements for everyone to read. (You can also photocopy some pages from this book.)

- ✔ **Let your loved ones understand that you're nothing if not serious about the lifestyle changes you're going to make.** (Well, aren't you?) But have a sense of humor about it. Don't make it sound as though you're going to do yourself in if your family doesn't do what you want them to do.

The most important points to convey include the following:

- ✔ What hypoglycemia is

- ✔ The importance of regulating your blood sugar

- ✔ How the wrong foods can contribute to your condition

- ✔ The health impact of a blood sugar imbalance

- ✔ The food plan you need to follow

- ✔ Exercise and other lifestyle changes you want to make

Chapters 2, 6, and 8 provide the info everyone needs about the particular topics listed here.

If this list seems like too much to discuss, simply inform your family that you have hypoglycemia and you're making dietary changes. Then show them the list of foods you can and can't eat.

Helping your significant other cope

You may feel as if you need to brace yourself for the worst after you have the heart-to-heart with your partner. She may take it well. Or she may not. Either way, there are things you can do to make it easier for her to accept your blood sugar issue as a legitimate illness and to help her better cope with the dietary and lifestyle changes that are ahead of you.

The following can help you help your significant other:

✔ **Be open and willing to answer any questions she may have.** Your partner is bound to have many questions. You're setting the right tone by addressing any concerns she may have, and demonstrating that you value her perceptions.

✔ **Talk to each other regularly.** Good communication is the key to making a relationship work. When you encounter a major life change, you have to negotiate the transition by discussing any issues that come up.

✔ **Regardless of what comes up, never blame your partner for what ails you.** Blame is a good way to kill good will in anyone, especially someone close to you. By staying neutral and non-judgmental, you're more likely to get your partner's understanding and cooperation.

✔ **Take responsibility for your own condition.** You may find yourself getting cranky or depressed because of your blood sugar imbalances. Be sure to apologize and make amends when you're feeling more stable. Doing so ensures that your partner is more willing to support you during your difficult times.

✔ **Try not to take anything too seriously.** Schedule lots of fun time together. Find the humor and the silver lining in any situation.

Talking to Your Children about Hypoglycemia

Your partner isn't the only person who should be informed about your metabolic syndrome. Children can sense when a parent is sick — hiding your condition from them isn't fair. You probably can't anyway, because you'll need to change your diet and make other adjustments that may have your children wondering what's going on.

This section provides some helpful ways to talk to your children and help them understand that your condition isn't life threatening.

Keep it simple

Even with adults, you need to keep things simple. Naturally, with children, keeping your explanations as simple as possible is even more important, because they may not be able to grasp the complexity of a health issue such as hypoglycemia. Don't hide your discomfort behind technical terms. View things from the perspective of a child.

Children have a shorter attention span than adults, so avoid long-winded explanations. Drawings and other visual aids are especially effective for children.

Be prepared for questions

Children are very curious (as if you didn't already know!) and will likely pepper you with questions. Answer every question to the best of your ability. It's important that children understand exactly what's going on with your health. Otherwise, they may become prone to anxiety and may let their imagination get the best of them.

When answering their questions, keep the following in mind:

- ✔ **Don't patronize and don't minimize their fears.** Children hate being talked down to. And when you shush them and discount their fears, they're likely to become even more afraid. Simply tell them that you're going to eat a healthier diet because you want to be healthy to take better care of them.

- ✔ **Address every concern your children may express.** Don't get angry or snap at them if they're resentful that they don't get to eat "fun" foods anymore. Tell them that they'll still get to enjoy some of their favorite foods, but it'll be healthier for the family to gradually change the diet so that everyone can be healthy and energetic. Because hypoglycemia isn't a life-threatening condition, don't make it a big deal.

- ✔ **Be specific and clear.** Don't use medical jargon that they don't understand. Use plain English. If an older child wants to understand more, you may be able to explain blood sugar mechanisms. But for a very small child, keep it very simple. All you have to say is that you'll be eating more vegetables and staying away from sweets.

Reiterate that they didn't make you sick

Some children may have a natural tendency to believe that they caused their parents' illnesses. Let them know that nothing they do can cause any kind of illness, including hypoglycemia. The fact that your body has a faulty mechanism for balancing blood sugar properly isn't their fault.

If you've been moody or depressed because of the hypoglycemia, say something like this: "I'm sorry, it's not your fault that I've been feeling ill/unhappy. It's not because you're bad that I've been so irritable with you. My doctor told me it's because I have low blood sugar. Now I'm changing to a healthier diet, and these problems I've had will go away."

Involving the Whole Family

Your family may ask you right off the bat what they can do to help. Naaaah! That would never happen, right? Asking for help from the people you love most (and who love you most) rests on your shoulders.

This section approaches the different ways you can talk to your family about your hypoglycemia, how you can get your family to help you deal with your hypoglycemia, and how your family can help with mealtime.

Can we talk?

If you want to involve the whole family, you have to talk. Set aside a time to talk. Make the occasion relaxing by pouring some herbal tea and playing soft music. Tell your loved ones that you want to have a heart-to-heart talk about an important matter.

✓ **Embrace your sweetheart or family members and make up for whatever nasty behavior your hypoglycemia caused.** Maybe you've let your significant other feel very much insignificant.

- Explain that a lot of the bad things — outbursts, fights, and misunderstandings — were due to the effects of low blood sugar.

- Accept full responsibility for your actions.

✓ **Get your loved ones to understand the sincerity of your intentions to redirect your lifestyle.**

✓ **Get your loved ones to understand your hypoglycemia.**

- Teach them about hypoglycemia and faulty glucose metabolism.

- Read them passages from this book.

- Create a list that describes who you are and what you're going through as you deal with your hypoglycemia (see Chapter 12 to become better acquainted with yourself, and then use that info to talk to your loved ones). Sometimes people understand written things better.

Helping your loved ones help you

Changing your diet and entire lifestyle isn't easy. Don't make it more difficult on yourself by being a lone ranger. Getting practical and emotional support from your family and friends can make your recovery easier. But sometimes those near and dear to you just don't understand that you need their help. You have to reach out and ask for the help. When they understand what you're striving for and why, they're more likely to be on your side.

Keep the following in mind when asking your family and friends for help:

- ✔ **Ask yourself first what your family can do to help.** (Either that or ask what you can do for your country.) Certain household chores may become difficult for you to do, for example, when hypoglycemia is paired with other syndromes like fibromyalgia.

- ✔ **State your requests clearly and in a matter-of-fact way.** For example, you're the cook, but you find that brain fog interferes with your duties. Give explicit instructions for someone else to make out a shopping list for you. Make meal planning a joint, cooperative venture.

- ✔ **Don't turn requests into threats or demands.** At the same time, don't sound apologetic.

- ✔ **If stress is a problem — and it usually is — figure out how you can tackle it together.** Brainstorm ways to deal with this and other issues.

- ✔ **Use "I" statements.** Statements that begin with "I" instead of "you" sound less like accusations. For example, suppose you're hurt because your spouse refuses to support you. You shouldn't say, "You're a real moron for not understanding how important this is to me. You always were a &%*$ [fill in with any of your favorite four-letter words]." A far better approach is, "I feel hurt when you won't listen to my explanations about how food can seriously affect my body chemistry and my ability to function. I tell myself then that you don't care about my health."

- ✔ **Don't interrupt, bring up unrelated elements, or change the subject.** Setting ground rules can go a long way toward smoother communication.

✔ **Use any digressions to get back to the main point.** Digression can bring up significant issues. For instance, when you're trying to communicate the frustrations you experience with hypoglycemia, and your partner complains that you never come through with your promises, you have the chance to point out that your failure to follow through is related to your particular biochemical disorder, and now that you know what's causing these problems, you're bound and determined to change them — and you need all the support you can get. Repeat or paraphrase what your loved one just said. This approach is also useful if you suffer from brain fog and tend to space out what someone's saying. Some digressions may lead to a whole different conversation. In that case, write it down and promise to talk about it later. Set aside a specific time to discuss the issue to make it clear that you're not simply making excuses to avoid the subject.

✔ **Don't keep your problem to yourself.** You may think that keeping your hypoglycemia to yourself will ensure harmony, but in the long run, this plan can backfire. Rather than let health problems create difficulties in your relationships, use them as a communication bridge to build a stronger foundation.

✔ **Express appreciation for any support your family gives you.** Giving thanks for specific acts of consideration is also a good idea. For instance, you may want to say, "Timothy, I really am thankful that you agreed to do all the grocery shopping for us. It helps me avoid foods I'm not supposed to have."

✔ **Express the love you feel.** Don't bottle it up; spread it around. Show love to your family and friends every day. Spend time having fun with them. Doing so works wonders with keeping your body chemistry balanced.

When can we eat?

Family functions often center on food. Think of the major holidays and special events from your life: cake on your birthday and turkey on Thanksgiving, not to mention all those summer barbecues and late-night pizzas. Then you have the daily grind. Someone has to cook dinner. Mac and cheese, anyone?

After talking with your family about what you're experiencing, tell them what you need in terms of food. For more information about food and diet, check out Chapter 6. In the meantime, try these tactics:

✔ Tell your family that you need to eat certain foods, avoid some foods, and eat frequently.

✔ Explain that you need their help in sticking to your food plan. Their help may involve reminding you to eat at appropriate times or helping with the preparation of the proper foods.

✔ Let them know what you don't want from them. For instance, you don't need anyone to lay a guilt trip on you.

✔ Write down a list of items for your diet and go grocery shopping with your spouse or other willing family members.

✔ If you're not the house chef, sit down with the cook and explain all your dietary requirements. Make a copy of your requirements so that the cook can refer to them easily. You can also offer to take turns cooking, if you aren't already doing so. Or you may want to cook together sometimes.

Do you have kiddies? Use this time to wean them off junk foods. They'll probably moan about not being able to eat the foods that all their friends are eating. However, don't force them to give up everything they like. As long as the bulk of their meals are wholesome, and they don't have special health problems requiring a particular diet, you shouldn't be overly strict. Simply stick with your own diet. When you become fit, strong, and energetic — and more balanced emotionally — they may become so impressed that they'll want to follow the example you set.

So you've created a food plan and now you're talking to your family about the do's and don'ts of the hypoglycemically correct diet. What better time to also discuss the when's of eating — in other words, good times for you to munch. If you're like most hypoglycemics, you'll have to eat fairly often — and you'll always need to have a snack within easy reach. Or, conversely, you may be the minority who has to space your meals apart carefully and not eat too frequently in order to stay symptom-free. Either way, planning is essential. And getting the understanding, if not the help, of your family is a good idea. You may try writing up an eating schedule and taping it to the kitchen wall as a reminder for everyone. (And carry a copy of it with you for easy referral.) When everyone is on the same page, sticking to the timetable is much easier.

When your loved one won't help

What if your spouse won't cooperate with your food needs? Well, for starters, you may want to consider couples counseling! Meanwhile, get some help from good friends and a support group. Consult an online hypoglycemia support group (see Chapter 12) for suggestions on what you can do when family members won't help. You may also want to use your support group for developing relationships.

You can change cooking from a chore to a big, fun family affair. One family, for instance, planned everything so that they could cook enough food to last an entire month. (Hey, what are freezers for?) They chose a day when they could all go grocery shopping together. When they finished shopping, they lugged a humongous amount of food to the car. They went wild the following day, cooking batch after batch of wonderful food. Everyone chipped in, including the kids.

If you shudder at the thought of preparing a month's worth of meals, you can fix food for a few days or a week or two. When hunger comes knocking at the door (actually, it shouldn't if you eat regularly like you're supposed to), you won't be tempted to gnaw at the forbidden when you have a delectable and healthy meal readily available.

Dealing with the Doubting Thomases

It's a fact of life. People may give you grief about your condition. Many people don't believe that diet and nutrition can have such a profound effect on someone with a sensitive body chemistry. Such people may think you're off the wall. They may even accuse you of malingering.

We want to say "Tough it out. Pump up your emotional defense muscles. Deflect the verbal punches." But that's much easier said than done, especially when you're feeling out of balance.

Although you may encounter a few doubters, you don't have to feel any more pain because of their negative responses. This section helps you stay clear of their negative behavior, avoid any unneeded conflict, and figure out how to protect yourself.

Staying clear of negativity

The best way to deal with doubting Thomases? Don't listen to them. When possible, avoid negative exchanges with doubters or other unsupportive people. Those exchanges can drive you back to emotional eating habits, which can trigger or aggravate your symptoms.

The following can help you:

- **Stop them in their tracks.** Refuse to discuss hypoglycemia or related topics with them. You can't convert someone with a heated exchange.

✔ **Switch the subject.** You can't and won't convert or convince someone with a heated exchange, so change the subject. If the doubter persists, be firm in telling him that you don't care to discuss it with him.

✔ **Have some fun with them.** You don't have to defend yourself. Instead of letting doubters get on your nerves, quibble over absolute irrelevancies, throw back non-sequiturs, recite nonsense poems, and confuse the heck out of them. As the saying goes, if you can't say anything nice, say something surreal.

If your family members give you grief when you speak to them about changing your diet, they may be feeling threatened by the prospect of change. You're tampering with diet and nutrition, the very foundation of family life — daily meals! If your family's eating habits are less than healthy, the prospect of change may trigger feelings of anxiety or guilt. The best remedy is to offer as much love and reassurance as you can. It may help to point out that you'll be a calmer, happier, more loving person as your blood sugar becomes better regulated and more balanced.

If you're without kith or kin, or your family simply doesn't support you, seek support elsewhere. Find advocates on your behalf and create a support network for yourself. (Flip to Chapter 12 for suggestions on setting that up.) Whenever possible and practical, get together with those in your support network to chat, share meals, and so on. Perhaps you can even host a get-together in your own home.

Avoiding conflict

You shouldn't be afraid of conflict; it's unavoidable in any relationship. You need to figure out how to work through disputes in a healthy manner.

Avoiding those you don't care about is one thing. With those whose lives are closely intertwined with yours, however, wanting to explain your side of the story is reasonable. If you're unable to resolve differences, however, take these tips to task:

✔ **Let it slide.** The best you can do in such cases is to agree to disagree.

✔ **Choose your battles carefully.** Conserve your energy for getting well. The erratic blood sugar syndrome may have drained you of energy or left you feeling out of control, scrambling to put the pieces of your life together.

✔ **Show consideration for others.** Showing consideration helps avoid misunderstandings or disagreements. In the case of social situations, such as dinner invitations, you can show consideration by alerting your host or hostess in advance. (Check out Chapter 16 for more details.)

Maintaining your boundaries

When the poet Robert Frost wrote that good walls make good neighbors, he was presenting sensible advice on living. By erecting a wall (literally as well as figuratively), you ensure that your neighbors respect your privacy and refrain from sticking their noses in your business. Just as a wall around your house protects you from prying eyes and trespassers, maintaining healthy emotional and mental boundaries prevents people from meddling in your affairs and keeps them from getting unwanted control of you.

Having healthy boundaries also means that you don't let other people's doubts seep into your consciousness, undermining your commitment to your recovery.

One man's ham

Katie, an American expatriate living in Tokyo, is a vegetarian who prefers to eat whole, natural, healthy foods. Finding restaurants in Japan that serve vegetarian fare is very difficult, so she compromises when eating out with people. One evening she went to a restaurant with a group of friends. She ordered a bowl of noodles that the waitress assured her didn't contain meat. When the noodles were brought to her table, however, they were swimming in greasy meat — too much for her to pick aside. She therefore reminded the waitress that she didn't eat meat and sent the bowl back to the kitchen. When the waitress brought back some more noodles, they were smothered with strips of ham. At that point, Katie and her friends left the restaurant without paying for their food, which they hadn't touched.

Being hungry and crabby (with their blood sugar plummeting, no doubt), they hurled insults at the restaurant staff before taking off. The incensed cook chased them down, grabbed the most defenseless-looking woman, and beat her down. The women called the police, who then forced them to pay for their meals. Why? According to the policeman, the restaurant had acted in good faith by serving them a vegetarian dish. Ham, he pointed out, isn't meat. Food that's generally accepted as vegetarian in Japan differs from what Westerners regard as vegetarian.

When in doubt — particularly if you're surrounded by hostile people — don't press the issue. Nibble on your snack if you're hungry and don't waste time arguing.

Boundary violations occur when people

- Tell you what you ought to be feeling

- Tell you what you ought to eat (unless they're medical professionals)

- Tell you how to run your life

- Suggest that you have no right to feel the way you do

- Make you feel guilty for having needs

- Make you feel guilty for needing reasonable accommodations

- Wonder out loud why you're always this or that (sick or tired, for example)

- Put you down or insult you in any way

Notice all the "oughts"? They ought not tell you how to be! But you definitely ought to

- **Be honest with yourself.** Doing so helps you know very clearly what you need and what's destructive.

- **Let others know when you reach your limits or they trespass on your boundaries.** Be confident when expressing your limits and boundaries.

- **Set very clear limits regarding what you'll tolerate.** When others make demands on your time and energy that you can't comfortably honor because of your health issues, calmly tell them so (in no uncertain terms).

- **Offer choices when someone makes demands you can't honor comfortably.** One way to handle the demands of others is to give them a choice. For instance, you can say, "I can either take the kids to the ball game or cook dinner, but not both. Which do you want me to do?" Make sure that you provide a clear message that you want to do your share, but you can't be expected to do everything. You'll be leaving room to work out a compromise.

- **Watch your tone.** It's not so much what you say but how you say it. If you whine, people react negatively. If you sound uncertain, others question you. Be as confident and upbeat as you can. Make your requests sweet and simple. And smile.

Sabotaging the saboteurs

Your doubters and critics — inner and outer — try to sabotage your best efforts. You'll always find people who delight in criticizing you, tormenting you, and making you doubt that anything you do will ever improve your health. Or maybe they don't set out to destroy you, but they whine about everything. Either way, these people are negative because they're unhappy with themselves. Remember that their negativity has nothing to do with you or your blood sugar.

Others

Like alcoholics who discover that they need a different circle of friends if they're to stay sober, you may have to let go of some friendships that are no longer serving your purpose. Bad friends prod you to go off your food program or complain that you're no longer any fun because you don't wash down a whole chocolate cake with root beer, or chug-a-lug a jug of beer as you scarf down mashed potatoes and deep-fried chicken.

Here are some suggestions for what to do when your critics start harping on about your new lifestyle, and no amount of reasoning on your part makes a dent. These suggestions are by no means a staple of good communication. But they sure can be fun!

- Walk out of the room.

- Interrupt them repeatedly.

- Laugh hysterically and don't explain why.

- Keep saying that you don't understand, and ask them to repeat themselves until you wear them down.

- Agree with them wholeheartedly and continue doing what you have to do.

- Thank them for sharing.

- Pretend that they're not there.

- Insist that health is now your new priority, and simply end the discussion.

Yourself

If you're your own personal saboteur, get guidance on positive self-talk or cognitive therapy. These days you can find numerous good books and audio programs that teach you how to change habitual, negative, fear-based thinking into "real-based" thinking.

With this type of thinking, you don't repeat mindless positive affirmations. Rather, you use affirming but realistic statements to steer your behavior in a more productive direction. After you get the hang of it, you'll make radical changes in your thinking, which can help you better control your diet and improve your blood sugar balance.

Chapter 14

Suffering Along with Your Sweetie?

....

....

*I*f you're living with — or closely interacting with — a hypoglycemic, you know that it's not exactly what you'd call a
Sunday picnic in the park. You may have discovered that your
family member, aside from any admirable qualities he may pos-
sess, isn't exactly made of sugar, spice, and everything nice. He
may be the sweetest, most charming, and most considerate person
in the world one minute, purring along contentedly, and the next
minute, he may suddenly turn his fangs on you. Indeed, you may
wonder whether your family member isn't suffering from a Jekyll-
and-Hyde–type personality. You're right, in a sense.

Depending on how severe the symptoms are, a hypoglycemic is
probably taking quite a ride. He may be experiencing a roller
coaster of chaotic emotions and unpredictable mood shifts. Life
may have simply become unmanageable. If so, take heart. It can all
be turned around. If your loved one follows the eating program
outlined in this book, he will soon be restored to sanity. How soon
he finds relief from his symptoms depends on various factors, such
as age, body constitution, discipline, and so on. In most cases,
however, he can feel some relief after several weeks; you should
see major changes after several months.

Whether you're the spouse, lover, parent, child, or friend of a hypoglycemic, your support can make all the difference in the world.
This chapter shows how you can support him by improving your
knowledge about the disease, using productive communication,
joining your love in the preparation of food, and improving your

own eating habits. You can make recovery from this pernicious condition faster, smoother, and easier.

Introducing Mr. (or Ms.) Hyde

So you have a Hyde on your hands: Your loved one is lashing out, and you're bearing the brunt. You can run from Hyde, or you can remember that Jekyll is in there. You're already solidly on the road to showing support: You're here, aren't you?

This section shows you where to turn so you can better grasp your Mr. (or Ms.) Hyde's hypoglycemia. It also discusses Hyde's symptoms so you know what to expect.

Understanding Hyde's condition

To offer the right kind of support, a solid understanding of hypoglycemia is useful. As with any illness, the more knowledge you have, the better. For starters, you can

- ✔ **Read this book.** You aren't surprised, are you?
- ✔ **Check out other resources on hypoglycemia.** This book includes many Web sites and resources that provide more info. You can also find books at your local library or bookstore.
- ✔ **Talk to other hypoglycemics and their families.** Other people who've lived with the same situation you have can offer you tips, examples, and moral support in a way that no one else can. When you talk to someone who's suffered through similar problems, solutions or explanations offered can feel so much more real and immediate than reading the same thing in a book. Besides, you won't feel so alone or isolated.
- ✔ **Consult with knowledgeable healthcare practitioners.** Professionals can give you insight, as well as provide a medical perspective that you or others may have missed. And needless to say, consult with a healthcare practitioner to make sure that your loved one is truly suffering from hypoglycemia and not some other condition.
- ✔ **Discuss the disorder with the sufferer.** Communication is the key to resolving any difficulties, regardless of the problem. As with any health condition, hypoglycemia can create tension and misunderstandings.
- ✔ **Put on headphones and sing as loud as you can.** Okay, maybe not the best idea, unless you want to get the local dogs barking.

Pursuing these paths to knowledge can lead you directly into the gaping mouth of what you run up against during one of Hyde's horrible hissy fits: symptoms.

Identifying Hyde's symptoms

Recognizing the typical signs of low blood sugar is crucial to help-ing yourself and your loved one. Common symptoms (which we discuss in more detail in Chapter 3) include

- ✔ Irritation
- ✔ Mental confusion
- ✔ Temper outbursts
- ✔ Crying jags
- ✔ Forgetfulness
- ✔ Excessive yawning (despite adequate sleep)
- ✔ Suddenly and inexplicably falling asleep (even when not in bed!)

The number, frequency, and severity of symptoms differ for each individual. Some people may be only mildly affected by symptoms, but it's probably fair to say that, for most hypoglycemics, life is a constant battle. They often struggle to get going and keep going when the spirit is willing but the body is flagging. Far too many have paid the price in checkered careers, strained interpersonal relationships, and unfulfilled dreams. And you, too, as a family member, have paid the price. Fortunately, you can do something about the symptoms associated with hypoglycemia.

Knowing what to expect can lead you to talk with your family member about what she's going through. As you discuss the ways that you can make it easier for her to change her diet and anything else that may be impeding her progress, your supporting role becomes clearer. The road to recovery starts with communication.

Talking It Over

Your loved one may act like a beast when she's having an attack of low blood sugar, but remember that she's a human being, and so are you. Use your tongue and teeth to talk to each other, not to tear each other to shreds. Words can heal as much as they can hurt; you just have to know the right words to say. When some-one's acting out, knowing what to say and what not to say can help keep a volatile situation from getting out of control.

To help keep the dust down while your family member is calm, the following sections give you some specific steps for communicating with a hypoglycemic and some do's and don'ts for talking with a hypoglycemic who's attempting to overhaul her diet and possibly change her exercise and work habits, as well.

Starting with the four Rs

Talking with your loved ones is an easy enough skill to develop, but because it's not something you're likely to know instinctively, we offer you the four Rs.

You can put the four Rs into action by following these steps:

1. **Recognize that when your loved one has hissy fits, it's the low blood sugar talking.**

   Don't take hypoglycemic symptoms personally. When a person has a hypoglycemic episode, not enough sugar is getting into the brain. The first area of the brain to shut down is the *neocortex* (the "civilized" portion of the brain), where higher learning and thinking take place. (Check out Chapter 2 for more info.)

2. **Refrain from getting involved in the drama.**

   Avoid these things:

   - Criticizing
   - Reasoning with the person
   - Getting drawn into an argument

   Of course, if someone snaps at you or behaves in an inappropriate fashion, reacting negatively is only human. Delivering a comeback may feel most natural and satisfying in the heat of the moment, but you end up only frustrating yourself. Not only do you fail to accomplish anything, but you may also make the battle escalate.

3. **Respond with compassion.**

   The following sections tell you how to convey your supportive feelings to the sufferer.

4. **Remind the hypoglycemic to eat.**

   Offer high-quality snacks. The snacks should have some protein and complex carbs: a boiled egg or a stick of celery with nut butter, for example. Do *not,* under any circumstances, provide anything with sugar and refined flours. You can rule out sodas, pastries, cookies, and ice cream, among other common snacks. (See Chapter 6 for acceptable snacks.) Remember that even a small amount of sugar or simple carbs can trigger symptoms.

You can always walk away from the situation for awhile. After the dust settles and your loved one's blood sugar returns to normal (whatever her optimal level may be), she'll most likely apologize profusely. When the reconciliation begins, you can at last attempt to have a discussion. If you need to make a joint decision about something, this is the time to do it. Don't try to make important decisions when her brain has shut down from lack of fuel.

Giving these words the green light

People are apt to think of low blood sugar sufferers as lazy and undisciplined, or as hypochondriacs who dream up imaginary illnesses in a desperate bid for attention. Low blood sugar sufferers receive little, if any, sympathy or understanding — even from themselves! They're often met with blame, criticism, or irritation.

Hypoglycemia isn't all in the mind, however. Recognized or not, something is going on physiologically. Hypoglycemia isn't some unfortunate fad (such as a bad haircut) that people choose so that they can stand apart from the crowd or gain sympathy. No wounds or scars may be visible, but the suffering is all too real.

Because hypoglycemia is a legitimate condition, the sufferer needs you to offer encouragement, sympathy, and support. You can show your support in the following ways:

✔ **Become an advocate.** Your loved one needs you, especially during hypoglycemic attacks, when the person is unable to think clearly. (These attacks are usually a result of forgetting to eat.) Again, remind yourself that it's the low blood sugar, not the sufferer, that's the problem.

✔ **Point out to your loved one which symptoms have disappeared.** When hypoglycemics feel discouraged, feel that they aren't healing fast enough, or feel that their diet isn't working, forgetting how things used to be is easy. Because most people have a tendency to concentrate on the negative — or on the symptoms that they continue to have — they may not notice that some of their symptoms have disappeared. Encourage your loved one to fill out the self-questionnaire in Chapter 5 if she hasn't already done so. Keep a copy of her completed questionnaire so that you can refer to it from time to time and remind her of how she used to be (and of how far she's come).

✔ **Offer words of encouragement.** The following list includes some words of encouragement that you can give to someone who's working to control her hypoglycemia:

  • "You're on the right track."

  • "You're doing great."

  • "I'm so proud of you."

  • "You're so much better than you used to be."

- "Remember how you used to be? You've come a long way (baby)."
- "Have you noticed that you're no longer suffering from [insert specific symptom here]?"

Stopping negative talk

One big drawback to suffering from hypoglycemia is that it's just not widely understood. It doesn't seem quite as legitimate as some of the more serious illnesses or disorders, such as cancer or diabetes, particularly because the medical profession generally doesn't recognize it. Lab tests, discussed in Chapter 5, can't always give a proper diagnosis of hypoglycemia. Because hypoglycemia has such a vast array of puzzling symptoms, it can feel like an anything-goes, catch-all syndrome — hardly something to take seriously.

If you want to show that you care and that you understand the full ramifications of low blood sugar, avoid these negative statements:

- ✔ "Snap out of it."
- ✔ "Grow up."
- ✔ "You're crazy."
- ✔ "It's all in your head."
- ✔ "What's your problem?"
- ✔ "Why can't you be like everyone else?"

Low blood sugar or not, refrain from negative comments, because they may make the other person defensive, leading her to shut down communication. Negative comments definitely aren't for nurturing a relationship. But if you do slip, don't be hard on yourself. The vast majority hasn't achieved sainthood yet, so just apologize and let it go. Don't let yourself engage in an escalating battle of blame.

Keep in mind that making dietary and lifestyle changes is difficult. You're bound to experience plateaus and what may appear to be setbacks. Low blood sugar sufferers — who are probably prone to be sensitive anyway — may feel quite discouraged.

To get everyone in the family on the same page, you may consider calling a family meeting. Lay down some basic do's and don'ts, such as comments that should be avoided or things that family members can do to support the hypoglycemic person. Make sure that no one in the family makes comments such as these:

✔ "C'mon, one bite won't hurt you." (No, but it can trigger a full-blown binge.)

✔ "Just start tomorrow." (And tomorrow and tomorrow . . .)

✔ "It's a holiday." (Or your birthday, or your anniversary, or the first day of the rest of your life. . . . The body doesn't care what occasion it is.)

✔ "What are you being so strict for? You don't need to lose weight." (The diet isn't about losing weight.)

✔ "You'll get sick if you don't eat." (Eating the wrong foods will make hypoglycemics sick, too.)

✔ "What a scrumptious dessert!" (It's nothing compared to the scrumptiously debilitating side effects the hypoglycemic will get from eating it.)

✔ "Don't tell me you're still trying to follow that crazy diet!" (What's crazy is the persistence of eating foods that cause distress to the hypoglycemic's metabolism — not to mention his life.)

✔ "What are you, some kind of health nut?" (Would you say that to a diabetic who has to watch his diet?)

Offering Your Offspring Support

As a parent, it's up to you to figure out whether your child is hypoglycemic. Children can't be expected to accurately fill out the self-survey questionnaire (see Chapter 5) for themselves. Observe your child closely. Answer the questions on his behalf.

If your child shows symptoms of low blood sugar, consult a physician. (Chapter 3 gives a list of common symptoms. Flip to Chapter 4 for advice on choosing a healthcare professional.)

Keep in mind these do's and don'ts when giving your child (or grandchild) support with his hypoglycemia:

✔ **Do encourage your child to stay on track.** Children may need more encouragement than adults to stay on a particular diet and nutrition plan. Cutting out excess sugar and fat, and junk foods in general, may be very difficult.

✔ **Do make the changes gradually.** Offer lots of love and support. Never threaten or belittle him, or make him feel like hypoglycemia is somehow his fault. It isn't.

✔ **Do reward your child.** Give children non-food rewards for sticking to the plan. Once in a great while, it may be okay to go off that plan as a special treat. Use your best judgment based on your child's particular situation.

✔ **Don't assume that your child will eventually grow out of it.** If you leave the dysfunction uncorrected, it's liable to get worse. Low blood sugar in a child's formative years can be even more damaging than blood sugar imbalance in an adult. Symptoms of hypoglycemia may impair your child's ability and motivation to learn and do well in school.

✔ **Don't make a hypoglycemic child feel isolated, different, or "afflicted."** Explain why good eating habits are important. Find healthy snacks the child can enjoy. (Flip to Chapter 6 for some suggestions.) Find the time to bake some healthy desserts for him if at all possible. It can boost morale enormously if everyone in the family follows a (mostly) hypoglycemic diet. A hypoglycemia-aware diet can be very healthy for everyone in the family, with only a few adjustments here and there for individual differences among family members.

Jumping In with Both Feet (and 2.5 Kids, a Dog, and a Cat)

The lifestyle changes in this book can benefit anyone. Today, most everyone suffers from stress and requires some form of exercise, and no one can function forever without proper rest and relaxation. Having a low blood sugar sufferer in your family (or your circle of friends) may be just the wake-up call you need. Take this opportunity to review your life, your diet, and your priorities.

Easy does it

Hey, don't let the prospect of a "lifestyle review" overwhelm or intimidate you. Even one or two small changes can work wonders when you consistently and diligently apply them. Whatever you do, have compassion, both for yourself and for the sufferer of low blood sugar. Just don't stress yourself out even more in a Herculean attempt to change everything at once. Easy does it.

Think of ways to make lifestyle changes pleasurable instead of treating them like chores or duties. For example, have fun, spend time with your family, and get a good workout by engaging in a group outdoor activity such as hiking or cycling. Or you can motivate both yourself and the person with hypoglycemia by buddying up with him and exercising together. (Flip to Chapter 8 for more about exercise and its benefits.)

Turn the healing and recovery project into a family affair. That may bring you closer together and enable the affected person to recover that much more quickly. For example, assign someone to remind the hypoglycemic to eat regularly every one-and-a-half to two hours.

Here are some other possible ways to get the family involved:

- ✔ **Openly discuss your feelings, especially if you have any concerns or reservations.** Do you feel threatened? Criticized? Made to feel wrong? Share what you think and how you feel among your friends and family, especially including others who also suffer from low blood sugar.

- ✔ **Turn the challenge of making dietary and lifestyle modifications into a game.** The way back to health doesn't have to be solemn, painful, hard work. Brainstorm with family and friends about ways to make the changes more fun, and therefore easier to stick to.

  For example, you may have a drawing or lottery to determine who does the different cooking and household chores. Or whip up new recipes that fit into your new diet and nutrition plan. Be creative! If you have kids, don't leave them out.

- ✔ **Show solidarity and support, but don't let the hypoglycemic act like a drama queen.** If she does flaunt an air of unspeakable sorrow, gently remind her that everyone has a cross to bear, but you're happy to help share some of the burden.

- ✔ **Have a sense of humor.** Take the journey to health with humor, and take it as lightly as you can, but don't pull a long face and become morbidly serious.

Family members often resist change out of ignorance or fear. This resistance is very natural, and very human. Be as supportive as possible to help everyone adapt to the situation.

You Be Betty Crocker and I'll Be Julia Child

When you live with a hypoglycemic, mealtime can't be slapdash or free-form. Don't just veg out in front of the TV with a bag of chips. And you shouldn't just order a pizza (although you can make a healthier homemade version).

To help make mealtime less stressful, we suggest you try the following:

✔ **Make shopping for and cooking healthy food a family affair.**
Eating junk food is never a good idea. You have to put more
thought into cooking and grocery shopping. Adults can take
turns shopping and cooking for healthy food. If you have children, they can contribute according to their age and ability.

✔ **Establish a regular routine.** Figure out a schedule for performing all meal-related activities, such as buying groceries (you
may see whether you can have the groceries delivered if that
makes life easier), freezing appropriate food items, and cooking. Also establish who's responsible for what. Write out everything on paper (try using a spreadsheet) and put it in the
kitchen or somewhere easily visible and accessible. After you
create and settle into a routine, meal preparation shouldn't take
an unusually long time. Meals and meal preparation can be fun
if everyone in the family pitches in.

✔ **Serve meals on a regular schedule.** Otherwise, your family
member's blood sugar may drop too low, and you may have
one easily upset person as a result.

✔ **Have everyone in the family eat the same healthy food.**
Adopting the same changes makes everything so much
simpler — not to mention healthier — for the whole family!

Of course, you don't have to eat as frequently as the hypoglycemic. You may want to stick to three average-size meals,
and maybe one snack. Note that average-size meals aren't
restaurant-size portions of food, which are typically too large.
You most likely share just one or two meals a day with the res-
ident hypoglycemic. (If you don't suffer from low blood sugar,
you don't have to restrict your carb intake quite as much. You
can consume 50 to 60 percent of your daily caloric intake in
the form of complex carbs.)

✔ **If you, the non-hypoglycemic, decide to occasionally eat
foods that are off limits to your loved one, don't flaunt it.**
Don't eat off-limit foods too often, and don't do so in front of
the hypoglycemic. Remember, tempt not, taunt not, flaunt not.
Your beloved hypoglycemic will appreciate your consideration, and you'll likely enjoy peace of mind. Do unto others as
you would have them do unto you. Changing your diet and
sticking to a nutrition plan is hard enough without having
temptation thrust in your face!

✔ **Be creative and ingenious.** Use your imagination to find
arrangements that work best for all concerned. If you're
adamant about sticking to your own diet, plan as much as
possible for some common mealtime together. For example,
everyone needs healthy helpings of greens, so include greens
(lots of greens!) among the dishes you both eat.

Part V
The Part of Tens

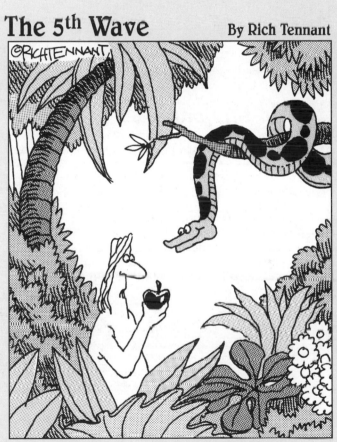

The 5th Wave   By Rich Tennant

"Well, yes, my blood sugar is a little low..."

In this part . . .

In this part, you find out what to do when temptation strikes. You discover how to better regulate your blood sugar, and you figure out what to do when you hit a snag. We dispel ten myths that surround hypoglycemia and give you ten hints to help you deal with your condition. Soon, you'll be ten times better than you ever were!

Chapter 15

Ten Myths about Hypoglycemia

Hypoglycemia is a condition that many doctors don't completely understand. In fact, some doctors even think that hypoglycemia isn't a real disease. Despite all the misunderstandings about hypoglycemia, the condition is real. (You know it if you suffer from it, right?)

This fun chapter debunks some common myths and misconceptions people have about hypoglycemia. Arm yourself with this info the next time some nonbeliever questions your condition.

Hypoglycemia Doesn't Exist

The truth is that hypoglycemia is a very real condition — all too real, in fact, for anyone who suffers from it. It should be taken seriously and treated just like any other health issue. People who assert that hypoglycemia doesn't exist or who use a definition that's too narrow leave hundreds of sufferers out in the cold.

Perhaps "hypoglycemia" isn't the best term to use because you may not suffer from low blood sugar as defined by the medical profession. (The speed at which the blood sugar drops is just as important. Chapter 5 provides details on how to diagnose hypoglycemia.) Yet, despite what blood sugar measurements may indicate, the fact is that people are afflicted with physical and emotional symptoms characteristic of hypoglycemia. It isn't a "fad disease" or a bogus diagnosis.

If the word *hypoglycemia* seems to elicit a dismissive shrug or a look of disbelief from most people, then feel free to use more descriptive (if not necessarily more accurate) terms like *blood sugar imbalance caused by insulin dysfunction, carbohydrate intolerance syndrome,* or a *metabolic dysfunction precipitated by inappropriate carbohydrate ingestion.*

Hypoglycemics Lack Willpower

Even when people acknowledge that hypoglycemia is a physical disorder, because it isn't something that they can point at or see, they have a tendency to regard its manifestations as simply the result of your overactive imagination. If you have a headache or feel weak, shaky, or dizzy, people may suspect you of malingering, especially if you're too ill to work.

People with hypertension can't normalize their blood pressure simply by willing their blood pressure to drop. By the same token, no one can achieve good blood sugar or hormonal balance by dint of sheer willpower. But some people have an assumption that you should be able to turn off symptoms and discomforts — especially if they're of an emotional rather than physical nature — by the strength of your mind power.

That's not realistic, and it's simply not possible. But you *can* take control of your life by gradually changing to a better diet and making any adjustments that you need to live a healthier, happier life. (Check out Chapter 6 for how you can eat a better diet.)

Eating Sugar Is a Quick Fix

If you believe that eating sugar is a quick fix for hypoglycemia, we want to offer you a training course guaranteed to make you a millionaire in just three months working from your home. That's not a likely scenario. And thinking that sugar will cure the low blood sugar blues is just as fanciful.

But why can't you just eat sugar if you don't have enough of it circulating in your bloodstream? In fact, eating something sweet quickly elevates the blood sugar level. And in an emergency situation, that's exactly what's required. Diabetics suffering from hypoglycemic shock take glucose tablets, drink orange juice, or eat a piece of candy — anything to pump up the blood sugar as quickly as possible.

However, an emergency situation is vastly different than a day-to-day scenario. Living a healthy lifestyle is a totally different story. You simply can't recover from hypoglycemia and become truly healthy if you continue to eat sugar and simple carbohydrates. If you do, the same old tiresome symptoms will keep popping up on your screen like bad reruns. Instead, choose complex, slow-release carbohydrates over trigger-happy, simple starches to keep your blood sugar balanced. (Check out Chapter 6 for more info on eating a healthful diet.)

One Diet Fits All

A nutritional plan that says that everyone must eat exactly the same way all the time isn't a good plan. Each person has different requirements, although just about everyone can make positive changes in his or her nutritional plan.

Even for hypoglycemics, there isn't one optimal diet that will put your health back on track. Some people benefit from a low-carbohydrate, high-protein diet, while others do much better eating a high-carbohydrate, low-protein diet. People benefit from different eating plans because everyone has a unique biochemistry.

Additionally, many people suffer from not only hypoglycemia, but also other associated conditions. For example, people who are allergic to wheat have to stay away from all foods containing wheat. There are, however, some food commandments that everyone must follow. Check out Chapter 6 for all the details. Stay away from sugar in all forms. And eat your vegetables.

Eliminating the "Bad" Foods Is All You Have to Do

Some people think that all you have to do is cut out the foods that trigger an overproduction of insulin. By avoiding foods that jack up the blood sugar too quickly, you won't experience a calamitous drop in blood sugar — it may seem as if your immediate problems are resolved.

But without eating the right foods and getting the nutrients that you need, you won't experience optimal health or a sense of well-being that comes from radiant health. Over the long term, you may even discover some of your old symptoms returning.

Speaking of elimination, another, often overlooked, ingredient should be included in the diet for people with blood sugar imbalances: fiber. Fiber helps with regular bowel movements. It's important in the prevention of constipation, varicose veins, hemorrhoids, and possibly colon cancers. The recommended intake is 25 to 35 grams (some experts suggest going as high as 50 grams), but the average person gets only about 11 grams per day.

Adding the right supplements is beneficial too, particularly as you get older. (Chapter 7 has recommendations on what to take.)

You Can't Be a Vegetarian if You're Hypoglycemic

People often say that being a vegetarian isn't possible if you suffer from hypoglycemia. They're presumably thinking about the often-heightened requirement for protein. But if you happen to be a vegetarian, you can still get enough protein. You don't even have to worry about combining the right foods to get all the amino acids you need in one sitting. Just try to include the following in your diet:

- ✔ A wide variety of vegetables
- ✔ Nuts
- ✔ Seeds
- ✔ Unrefined grains
- ✔ Soy products. They make good meat substitutes, but don't try to meet your protein needs solely through soy. (Flip to Chapter 6 for more on soy.)
- ✔ Natto. These sticky, fermented beans are a great vegetarian source of protein that are also rich in B-12, a vitamin that's usually missing from the vegetarian diet. In Japan, natto is often eaten over rice for breakfast. The one drawback to natto is its strong odor, which takes some getting used to.

When you're buying imitation meat products, be sure you check the labels for MSG, because it can derail your recovery. And depending on the brand, imitation meat may contain more carbs than protein.

Having a "Cheat Day" Is Okay

Some people ask about having a "cheat" day — a day you can go off your diet and eat anything you want. Because the hypoglycemia diet is designed to correct and prevent blood sugar imbalance, a day where you go off the diet doesn't make much sense. Unless of course you want to have a day where you throw progress to the wind and experience the joys of your body going haywire again.

 After you have a solid recovery, you can occasionally eat foods that are on the forbidden list. But an entire day where you eat anything you want at all will likely make you very ill.

If you just have to have sweets, make sure you eat some protein with them to slow down the sugar's entry into your bloodstream. And make sure that you're exercising enough — studies have shown that exercise can help reduce cravings for sugar.

Sugar Can Be Part of a Healthful Diet

Sugar can and is part of many people's diet — in fact, the vast majority of people in developed countries eat sugar. But it most definitely can't be a part of a *healthful* diet. Humans (some individuals more than others) are genetically predisposed to like sweet taste. But people aren't genetically built to consume several tons of sugar a year. Nor are humans pre-programmed to require an infusion of cookies or cream-filled cakes.

 Sure, a little bit of sugar won't kill you. When you're in good health, you can occasionally eat some sugar now and then, but you probably won't even like sweets the way you used to. You have to watch out if you're a sugar addict, because even a little bit can hook you back in. Saying that a little bit of sugar is okay is like telling an alcoholic that one drink won't hurt him.

If you continue to have cravings for sugar and other foods that are off limits, you may be deficient in one or more nutrients. For example, a craving for chocolate may indicate a lack of magnesium. Refer to a table created by Dr. Colleen Huber showing what you may be missing and what foods or supplements you can take at www.naturopathyworks.com/pages/cravings.php.

Hypoglycemics Should Eat Low-Fat Diets

For most people, eating an extremely low-fat diet is difficult to sustain and may lead to overeating. Fat is particularly important to anyone prone to low blood sugar. As Dr. Carolyn Dean, a physician who treats patients with chronic conditions, explains, "Sugar and fruit burn like paper; complex carbs burn like kindling; but fats burn like coal — lasting the longest and keeping your blood sugar up."

Dropping fat to lower than 20 percent of your total calorie intake makes sustaining balanced blood sugar and athletic performance more difficult. For most people, somewhere between 20 to 40 percent is the right range. Rather than the amount of fat, what you should be concerned about is the kind of fat you're eating.

Experts advise getting a variety of different oils. Try to get some monosaturates, like olive oil, and polyunsaturates, like flax oil. Omega-3 fatty fish oil is particularly relevant to anyone with blood sugar issues because the oil has a direct impact on how sensitive the cells are to insulin.

The fats that cause the greatest problems are *trans fats,* or partially hydrogenated oil. Trans fats appear in most packaged foods and are often lurking in restaurant foods. So how much trans fats do you need? Zero to none. Better cook at home, because most people get their trans fats from restaurants.

Don't be misled by labels that claim no trans fats. The ingredients may show some hidden trans fats. Even small amounts can quickly add up.

Blood Glucose Levels Remain the Same throughout the Day

Many patients think that blood sugar levels are the same no matter what time of the day it is — and that, moreover, they have to ensure that their glucose levels stay exactly the same all the time. In fact, everyone's blood sugar level has normal variations. Your aim is to keep your blood sugar fairly stable and avoid wide swings that can cause uncomfortable symptoms. But you can't — and don't need to — attempt to eliminate normal fluctuations in glucose levels.

 You'll find that your blood sugar is at the lowest before meals — this is why doctors urge hypoglycemics to eat frequently, and not go longer than three hours between meals and snacks. You should also eat a small snack before going to bed so your blood sugar doesn't drop too low in the middle of the night. To avoid weight gain, keep the calories low.

Chapter 16

Ten Hints for Helping Hypoglycemics

● ●

In This Chapter
▶ Making changes to your diet and lifestyle
▶ Improving the performance of your brain

● ●

Maybe you're feeling like a sourpuss because, when it comes to hypoglycemia, you have so much to be careful about. Dealing with hypoglycemia may seem daunting, but it's nothing you can't handle. You'll see for yourself that "doing" is indeed easier than "thinking about doing."

With the tips compiled in this chapter, you don't have to be hyper-vigilant about your hypoglycemia. Besides, most of the dietary and lifestyle changes are good for you regardless of whether you have hypoglycemia.

Acting Practically at Home

Okay, so you have to work, eat, sleep, pay bills, do the laundry, and spend some quality time with those you love. Try to incorporate these things into what free time you have:

✔ **Keep a list of foods to eat and foods to avoid on the fridge.** Carry a copy of the list with you wherever you go so that you can refer to it often. Chapter 6 gives further food fodder.

✔ **Be prepared for emergencies.** Don't go anywhere without food. Keep utensils, paper towels, and several coolers in your car, or bring a tote bag full of snacks. Keep the coolers supplied with several days' worth of food when you go on road trips.

✔ **Review your food journal every week.** Make any necessary adjustments to your food plan. (Chapter 6 gives info on journaling.)

✔ **Ventilate your house.** If the air in your house is stagnant, stir it up with electric fans. You may also want to install an attic fan. Avoid using air fresheners.

Testing for Sugar

To eat or not to eat? Ah, what a dilemma! When eating out, you can't always tell whether a dish has sugar; the server may not know, either.

Diabetes expert Dr. Richard Bernstein recommends carrying some Clinistix or Diastix (available at most pharmacies) to detect the presence of sugar or flour in packaged or restaurant foods. They're actually marketed for testing urine — but not to fear, he's not asking you to pee right at the table. To use these test strips for testing food, follow these steps:

1. **Put a small amount of food in your mouth.**

2. **Swish it or chew it around a bit so that it mixes with your saliva.**

3. **Spit a tiny bit onto a test strip.**

   The strip will change color if your food contains sugar. The darker the color, the more sugar it contains. The test strips will work on nearly all foods except milk products, which contain lactose. They also won't react with fructose.

Your loved ones are probably so used to your strange rituals involving food that they won't even blink when you conduct this test. But if you're dining with business associates, perform the test in the bathroom or just skip it altogether and order only tried-and-true dishes. Grilled or broiled meat and fish are safe bets. You can order some steamed vegetables, or you can have salad with oil and vinegar (because most dressings contain sugar). If you can't have vinegar, sprinkle some lemon juice and a dash of salt on your salad.

Controlling Blood Sugar

Diabetics use glucose tablets to raise their blood sugar, but some low blood sugar sufferers report that glucose tabs help them, too. To keep your blood sugar from dipping too low, eat more frequently — and carry some snacks with you.

Use glucose tabs with discretion. Taking them may put you in danger of a rebound drop in blood sugar. In other words, your body may produce too much insulin in response to the sugar, which in turn can cause your blood sugar to fall too low. Carry the tabs with you in case of emergencies and use them only

- ✔ When you have very severe symptoms
- ✔ If you eat some protein within 20 minutes of taking them

Because glucose doesn't have to be digested, the tablets can raise your blood sugar rapidly with a predictable outcome. Dr. Bernstein recommends Dextrotabs because they're inexpensive, conveniently packaged, and very easy to chew. Dextrotabs begin raising your blood sugar in about 3 minutes and stop raising it after about 40 minutes.

One point to bear in mind is that even if your blood sugar isn't too low, you may still have symptoms of hypoglycemia, such as a rapid heart rate, anxiety, tremors, and so on. If you wait a bit, they should abate.

Refrain from consuming too much during meals or snacks to avoid triggering too large an insulin response, which plays havoc with your blood sugar regulation. If you often feel hungry even after a reasonable meal, try finishing your meal with something that contains fat, because it tends to satisfy your appetite more. You may have a few slices of avocado or salad with lots of dressing. (Read the labels! Many brands contain sugar.) Also, if you're constantly hungry, you may not be getting enough of the right nutrients. You shouldn't get so hungry if you're eating frequent snacks. Review your diet and take some vitamins. (Check out Chapters 6 and 7 for more.)

Dining Out: The Do's and Don'ts

Who doesn't eat out once in a while? Eating at a restaurant or a friend's home doesn't need to spell disaster. Although you can't have your cake and eat it too (no cake allowed on the food plan, unless it's homemade without sugar or refined flour), you can follow these simple guidelines to help manage your diet:

- ✔ About half an hour before going to a restaurant, eat a light snack. You never know how long you'll have to wait.

- ✔ Tell the server about your allergies, sensitivities, and dietary restrictions, and don't be afraid to request modifications or substitutions.

✔ Stay away from white rice, white bread, noodles, anything with sauces, chips, bean paste, barbecued meats, sweet and sour foods, meatloaf (it often contains sugar or sweetener), casseroles (no telling what ingredients are in them), and anything deep fried. (More on foods to avoid in Chapter 6.)

✔ Because you're now eating smaller meals, most restaurant servings will be too large. To prevent overeating, measure out the amount you're going to eat and put the rest away in a doggie bag. Most restaurants in the United States serve such humongous portions that you can easily get three meals out of a single entrée. Think of all the money you're saving!

✔ Try ordering several appetizers instead of an entrée. It's a fun way to create a balanced meal. When ordering soups, be aware that they may be loaded with sugar.

✔ When your friends invite you to dinner, make your restrictions known but be gracious about it. Don't insist that they accommodate you.

- Offer to bring a dish to share — something you can definitely eat.

- Refuse politely when your host urges you to eat something you can't.

- Don't be uncertain or apologetic.

- Don't moan about your food restrictions, or your host may feel compelled to talk you into eating things that are off-limits.

✔ If everyone's having dessert and you're tempted beyond reason, order a sweet fruit (or bring some with you).

- If it's winter and you're cold, get a cup of tea and sweeten it with stevia, a natural low-carbohydrate sweetener. Carry several packets with you. (Some hypoglycemics can't tolerate stevia, because it can lower blood sugar. Try it out at home and see whether your body can handle it.)

- If all else fails, and you have to have a "real" dessert, get a bite from someone or share an order.

✔ You may find that there are times, such as special occasions, when you just have to have forbidden foods. In this case, you can go off your program, but make sure that you

- Plan ahead — and be willing to pay the consequences.

- Don't go off your program at a stressful time in your life — stress can aggravate hypoglycemia.

- Don't go off your program for too long.

- Always eat some protein to offset any sugar and concentrated carbs that you may eat.

✔ When staying with friends or relatives over a period of time, you may be able to make special requests if you have a close enough relationship with them. Otherwise, do what you can without imposing. Chapter 6 tells you more about diet, and Chapters 13 and 14 tell you how to live with a hypoglycemic. No matter what, be a considerate, gracious guest.

Food Facts for Tasty Health

Research is turning up more hard-core data about just how good certain foods (of course, we're talking natural stuff, like veggies and fruits, not prepackaged edibles) can be for your mind and body. In some cases, food can work like medicine — and it's probably the best-tasting medicine there is! The following facts about food can help you create a healthier diet:

✔ **Unless you're cooking for an army, get smaller bottles of cooking oil.** Add a capsule of vitamin E to the oil to help prevent oxidation, and throw out any oil that's been sitting for more than four months.

✔ **Use potato flour, barley flour, arrow root flour, oat flour, rice flour, or kuzu for thickening (replacing cornstarch).** If you're allergic to corn, avoid cornstarch.

✔ **Definitely add milled flaxseed to your diet.** It promotes healthy sugar metabolism by slowing down sugar absorption. Its high fiber content helps keep you regular. It's also a boon to anyone at risk of type 2 diabetes. On top of that, it supports your immune system.

✔ **Remove starch from some of your favorite foods.** To remove some of the starch from potatoes, cut them up and soak them in water overnight, and then drain them. To remove some starch from your oatmeal, cook it in twice the amount of water required, and then pour it through a strainer.

✔ **Eat an apple (or onion) a day.** Anyone with a blood sugar disorder should heed this advice. Apples and onions are rich in *quercetin* (a *flavonoid,* potent antioxidants found in most plants), which lowers the risk of developing type 2 diabetes, stroke, lung cancer, heart disease, and asthma.

✔ **Eat more fruits (if you can tolerate them).** Fruits are good for you. The darkest fruits, such as black or red grapes, are the richest in antioxidants, which help detoxify the body. Berries are also packed with antioxidants.

✔ **Consume almonds and turkey.** They not only provide protein, but they're also excellent sources of vitamin B6. This vitamin plays an important role in the synthesis of *serotonin* (the neurotransmitter that makes you feel calmer and happier).

✔ **Toast some seaweed.** Toasted nori (seaweed), which is available in Asian markets, is high in nutrients and very low in calories. It's also good for sluggish thyroids. Eating kelp and seaweed daily for at least a month will help regulate your thyroid.

✔ **Enjoy some sweet taste without unduly raising your blood sugar.** Add protein shake powder to plain, full-fat yogurt, and sweeten with stevia, if you can tolerate this natural sweetener. Or mix fruit-sweetened jam with some creamed cottage cheese. Be sure to get yogurt and cottage cheese with active cultures, because they may help grow beneficial bacteria in your intestines.

Noshing on Nourishment

Vegetables make excellent nutrient-packed snacks. Make sure that you have a good supply of raw vegetables, such as broccoli, cauliflower, cucumbers, celery, and bell peppers, washed and cut into finger-sized pieces. For added flavor, dip them in red or white miso paste, or drizzle a little bit of salad dressing on them. You can make a healthy salad dressing by combining extra virgin olive oil with balsamic vinegar. Or try spreading nut butter, such as almond or cashew, on the vegetables. Although not conclusive, some research suggests that the unsaturated fats in nuts may help regulate blood sugar. However, be cautious about eating too much, because nuts are high in calories and can cause weight gain. Seeds are rich in protein, but somewhat less fattening than nuts. Some vegetables, nuts, and seeds that you may want to try are

✔ **Leafy vegetables (such as kale or collards):** These vegetables can be cooked very quickly. Put them in a pot with just enough water to cover them. Boil for 3 or 4 minutes. Drain and freeze individual portions in baggies.

You can also keep individual portions of leafy green salads (also rich in vitamin E) in the fridge for snacking. Don't add the salad dressing until just before you eat.

✔ **Salted green soybeans (edamame):** They're usually found frozen in Asian supermarkets. Cook them in boiling water for five minutes and drain. Cool them under running water before eating, or refrigerate and serve chilled.

✔ **Artichokes:** Steam or boil for about 45 minutes. You may want to try them with low-fat salsa or other dips you enjoy.

✔ **Brussels sprouts:** Like other members of the cruciferous family (like broccoli), they're thought to fight cancer. You can steam them, or boil them, covered, for eight to ten minutes, until they're slightly tender but still crisp.

✔ **Almonds:** They have vitamins that play an important role in the synthesis of serotonin, the neurotransmitter that helps you feel happy. Other good serotonin-boosters are tomatoes, eggplants, and walnuts.

✔ **Raw walnuts and pumpkin seeds:** These are great sources of Omega-3 fatty acids, which modern diets are very low in. If you get tired of eating plain, raw pumpkin seeds, try Pumpkorn (seasoned pumpkin seeds), found in natural food stores.

Eating Brainy Foods

Did you know that the brain is made up of 60 percent fat? No kidding! If that was your body fat percentage, you'd be considered obese! The following nutrients can help your gray matter:

✔ **Vitamin E:** The brain is susceptible to harmful *oxidation* (a process that damages cells and genes). Taking plenty of vitamin E helps slow down oxidation and reduce memory loss. Brussels sprouts and avocados are good sources of vitamin E.

✔ **Omega-3 fatty acids:** You can find Omega-3 fatty acids in fatty fish, such as salmon, sardines, herring, mackerel, and anchovies. They help your body build more brain cells. Eating fish three to four times a week not only boosts your brain power but also lifts your mood. If you're a vegan, take one or two teaspoons of flax oil five times a week. Flax oil is also rich in Omega-3, so use it instead of butter on your bread, or add it to your salad.

✔ **Folate:** Legumes and green vegetables hold lots of folate, which is a B vitamin. All the B vitamins are very important in brain development and cognitive health.

Banishing Brain Fog

The fog that just rolled in isn't outside the window. It's in your head. And the worst part is that because you can't think clearly, you can't quite figure out what to do. Fortunately, you can take action to alleviate the problem. Try the following suggestions and see whether one, or a combination of them, works for you:

✔ **Chew gum:** Chewing gum may stimulate and improve your short-term memory. Studies have shown an increase in the activity of the *hippocampus* (the area of the brain where new memories are stored) when people chew gum.

✔ **Use ozone air-purification machines regularly:** They're a boon to people who live or work in places with airborne pollutants, fumes, mold, mildew, and so on. You can get a portable machine for home use. You'll start to notice the benefits after two to three weeks.

✔ **Eat nutritious foods:** Nutritious foods not only enhance your memory and learning but they may also help dispel brain fog. Nutritious foods include most kinds of vegetables, fruits (if you can tolerate them), and some lean protein such as organic chicken and beef.

✔ **Kick caffeine:** It gives you a temporary buzz, but in the long-run, it aggravates your health condition. Rather than drinking coffee, you may want to try drinking the South American herb yerba mate, which can give you a lift without the coffee jitters.

✔ **Take oral DHEA (dehydroepiandrosterone):** If you can say the word five times without stumbling, your brain's doing pretty good! DHEA is a steroid hormone. The concentration of DHEA in the human body plummets as people age. Studies suggest that DHEA improves memory and increases physical and psychological well-being. A daily dose of 30 to 90 mg may enhance the brain's ability to process and store information.

✔ **Shake, shake, shake your bod:** Let all your limbs go loose and roll your head freely while breathing naturally. Do it for anywhere from one to five minutes. It's an old qigong exercise that helps you relax and sweep away any cobwebs from your mind. (Chapter 8 talks more about qigong.) Here's another exercise you can try:

   1. **Stand with your knees slightly bent and your feet shoulder-width apart.**

   2. **Bring your arms up, as if carrying a ball.**

      Your elbows should be rounded, and your palms should face you. Your right and left fingertips should almost touch.

   3. **Close your eyes and take a few deep breaths.**

      Imagine that you're standing in a waterfall. Water is running down your head, face, and body, clearing your mind and cleaning your body.

   4. **Do this exercise for five minutes to an hour.**

✔ **Exercise your hands:** One exercise you can try is "dry washing." All you have to do is wring your hands, as though you're washing them, for one to five minutes. You can also hold golf balls in your palms and then roll them with your fingers; or you can just go through the motions empty-handed.

✔ **Give yourself a pat on the face:** Here's an exercise adapted from the Luohan Patting System of Yin Style Bagua (a school of Chinese martial arts and healing). Don't hit yourself too hard! You don't need to use a lot of force, just make it rhythmical.

   1. **Using cupped palms, slap your head from the front to the back, and to the sides above your ears.**

   2. **Lightly strike your forehead, temples, and cheeks.**

   3. **Count 1-2-3, 1-2-3, 1-2-3-4, 1-2-3, and then pause slightly before repeating the sequence.**

      (Or you can repeat, "Hot cross buns, hot cross buns, 1-2-3-4, hot cross buns.")

✔ **Laugh:** Laughing out loud releases endorphins, which makes you more alert and clears that foggy feeling. You don't actually have to have anything to laugh about. Going through the motions of laughing can provide you with the same benefits.

Remembering How to Deal with Short-Term Memory Loss

The brain has a higher metabolic rate than other organs, so if it isn't getting enough oxygen, glucose, and other substances that the brain cells need to function, your thinking may get fuzzy. You may find yourself spending several hours every day looking for misplaced items or forgetting things that should be second nature to you, such as remembering to take your wallet with you.

The best way to deal with this short-term memory loss is to

✔ **Write down everything that's important.** Keep a written record for everything, such as credit card payments, health-care information, and so on.

✔ **Put lists everywhere.** Make sure that you place them someplace visible. Write appointments, messages, and reminders on a wall calendar and a day planner.

✔ **Give directions aloud.** You may want to make sure that you're alone — or else pretend that you're speaking to a cellphone. Repeat the info you want to remember out loud several times.

✔ **Keep important items somewhere visible.** Make sure that you place your medication and vitamins someplace where you can see them. If you have items that you want to take with you when you go out, put them in your car, in your bag, or by the door.

✔ **Keep everything well organized.** Go through files, drawers, and closets. Do you have so much clutter that you don't know where to begin? Hire a professional organizer. If money is an issue, get a friend or family member to help you.

✔ **Keep chores and errands to an absolute minimum.** Conserve your energy for the essentials: making sure that you're getting enough nutrients, eating small meals, and exercising.

Changing Successfully

First, you step into a phone booth, then you rip off your . . . No, not that kind of change. We're talking about modifying your behavior to attain a goal that's important to you. And you don't have to transform yourself into a superhero in the blink of an eye, or overhaul your lifestyle overnight.

The problem? Staying with the status quo is easier than changing a long-standing habit or trying something new. Fortunately, after studying human behavior, psychologists have outlined a course of action that helps most anyone change successfully.

What follows is a simplified version of steps you can take to make revising your diet and lifestyle easier:

✔ **Take baby steps.** Break down the *target behavior* (the new behavior that you want to develop) into smaller, self-contained units. For example, you can write down each step that's entailed in changing your diet to a healthy one. It may be to start keeping a food journal, shopping for the right foods, cooking more at home, and so on. Approach each step as a separate mission (smaller goals that work toward the ultimate goal) and reward yourself whenever you accomplish them.

✔ **Identify elements in your environment that interfere with your target behavior.** After identifying what helps and what hinders, keep or increase what helps, and eliminate anything that hinders.

✔ **Eliminate the wrong foods.** This step is crucial in getting over hypoglycemia. Some people may be able to go cold turkey by giving up all their favorite foods and overhauling their lives overnight. For most people, it's much easier to change in degrees. See Chapter 6 for more info on maintaining a good diet.

✔ **Write down the consequences of continuing your current behavior.** Then write down all the benefits of reaching your goal. When you have a concrete picture of the positive results the new behavior can bring, you'll be more motivated to change to a healthier lifestyle.

Index

BUSINESS, CAREERS & PERSONAL FINANCE

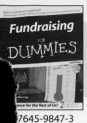

Fundraising For Dummies
0-7645-9847-3

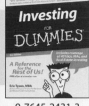

Investing For Dummies
0-7645-2431-3

Also available:

- Business Plans Kit For Dummies
  0-7645-9794-9
- Economics For Dummies
  0-7645-5726-2
- Grant Writing For Dummies
  0-7645-8416-2
- Home Buying For Dummies
  0-7645-5331-3
- Managing For Dummies
  0-7645-1771-6
- Marketing For Dummies
  0-7645-5600-2

- Personal Finance For Dummies
  0-7645-2590-5*
- Resumes For Dummies
  0-7645-5471-9
- Selling For Dummies 0-7645-5363-1
- Six Sigma For Dummies
  0-7645-6798-5
- Small Business Kit For Dummies
  0-7645-5984-2
- Starting an eBay Business For
  Dummies
  0-7645-6924-4
- Your Dream Career For Dummies
  0-7645-9795-7

HOME & BUSINESS COMPUTER BASICS

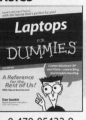

Laptops For Dummies
0-470-05432-8

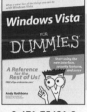

Windows Vista For Dummies
0-471-75421-8

Also available:

- Cleaning Windows Vista
  For Dummies 0-471-78293-9
- Excel 2007 For Dummies
  0-470-03737-7
- Mac OS X Tiger For Dummies
  0-7645-7675-5
- MacBook For Dummies
  0-470-04859-X
- Macs For Dummies 0-470-04849-2
- Office 2007 For Dummies
  0-470-00923-3

- Outlook 2007 For Dummies
  0-470-03830-6
- PCs For Dummies 0-7645-8958-X
- Salesforce.com For Dummies
  0-470-04893-X
- Upgrading & Fixing Laptops For
  Dummies 0-7645-8959-8
- Word 2007 For Dummies
  0-470-03658-3
- Quicken 2007 For Dummies
  0-470-04600-7

FOOD, HOME, GARDEN, HOBBIES, MUSIC & PETS

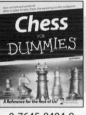

Chess For Dummies
0-7645-8404-9

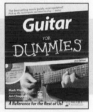

Guitar For Dummies
0-7645-9904-6

Also available:

- Candy Making For Dummies
  0-7645-9734-5
- Card Games For Dummies
  0-7645-9910-0
- Crocheting For Dummies
  0-7645-4151-X
- Dog Training For Dummies
  0-7645-8418-9
- Healthy Carb Cookbook For
  Dummies 0-7645-8476-6

- Home Maintenance For Dummies
  0-7645-5215-5
- Horses For Dummies 0-7645-9797-3
- Jewelry Making & Beading
  For Dummies 0-7645-2571-9
- Orchids For Dummies 0-7645-6759-4
- Puppies For Dummies 0-7645-5255-4
- Rock Guitar For Dummies
  0-7645-5356-9
- Sewing For Dummies 0-7645-6847-7
- Singing For Dummies 0-7645-2475-5

INTERNET & DIGITAL MEDIA

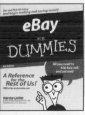

eBay For Dummies
0-470-04529-9

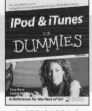

iPod & iTunes For Dummies
0-470-04894-8

Also available:

- Blogging For Dummies
  0-471-77084-1
- Digital Photography For Dummies
  0-7645-9802-3
- Digital Photography All-in-One Desk
  Reference For Dummies
  0-470-03743-1
- Digital SLR Cameras and
  Photography For Dummies
  0-7645-9803-1
- eBay Business All-in-One Desk
  Reference For Dummies
  0-7645-8438-3

- HDTV For Dummies
  0-470-09673-X
- Home Entertainment PCs
  For Dummies 0-470-05523-5
- MySpace For Dummies
  0-470-09529-6
- Search Engine Optimization
  For Dummies 0-471-97998-8
- Skype For Dummies 0-470-04891-3
- The Internet For Dummies
  0-7645-8996-2
- Wiring Your Digital Home
  For Dummies 0-471-91830-X

Separate Canadian edition also available
Separate U.K. edition also available

 WILEY

SPORTS, FITNESS, PARENTING, RELIGION & SPIRITUALITY

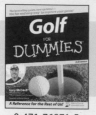

Golf For Dummies
0-471-76871-5

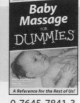

Baby Massage For Dummies
0-7645-7841-3

Also available:
- Catholicism For Dummies 0-7645-5391-7
- Exercise Balls For Dummies 0-7645-5623-1
- Fitness For Dummies 0-7645-7851-0
- Football For Dummies 0-7645-3936-1
- Judaism For Dummies 0-7645-5299-6
- Potty Training For Dummies 0-7645-5417-4

- Buddhism For Dummies 0-7645-5359-3
- Pregnancy For Dummies 0-7645-4483-7 †
- Ten Minute Tone-Ups For Dummies 0-7645-7207-5
- NASCAR For Dummies 0-7645-768?
- Religion For Dummies 0-7645-526?
- Soccer For Dummies 0-7645-52?
- Women in the Bible For Dumm? 0-7645-8475-8

TRAVEL

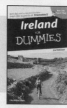

Ireland For Dummies
0-7645-7749-2

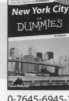

New York City For Dummies
0-7645-6945-7

Also available:
- Alaska For Dummies 0-7645-7746-8
- Cruise Vacations For Dummies 0-7645-6941-4
- England For Dummies 0-7645-4276-1
- Europe For Dummies 0-7645-7529-5
- Germany For Dummies 0-7645-7823-5
- Hawaii For Dummies 0-7645-7402-7

- Italy For Dummies 0-7645-7386-1
- Las Vegas For Dummies 0-7645-7382-9
- London For Dummies 0-7645-4277?
- Paris For Dummies 0-7645-7630-5
- RV Vacations For Dummies 0-7645-4442-X
- Walt Disney World & Orlando For Dummies 0-7645-9660-8

GRAPHICS, DESIGN & WEB DEVELOPMENT

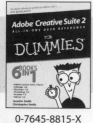

Adobe Creative Suite 2 All-in-One Desk Reference For Dummies
0-7645-8815-X

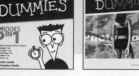

Photoshop CS2 For Dummies
0-7645-9571-7

Also available:
- 3D Game Animation For Dummies 0-7645-8789-7
- AutoCAD 2006 For Dummies 0-7645-8925-3
- Building a Web Site For Dummies 0-7645-7144-3
- Creating Web Pages For Dummies 0-470-08030-2
- Creating Web Pages All-in-One Desk Reference For Dummies 0-7645-4345-8
- Dreamweaver 8 For Dummies 0-7645-9649-7

- InDesign CS2 For Dummies 0-7645-9572-5
- Macromedia Flash 8 For Dummies 0-7645-9691-8
- Photoshop CS2 and Digital Photography For Dummies 0-7645-9580-6
- Photoshop Elements 4 For Dummie? 0-471-77483-9
- Syndicating Web Sites with RSS Fee? For Dummies 0-7645-8848-6
- Yahoo! SiteBuilder For Dummies 0-7645-9800-7

NETWORKING, SECURITY, PROGRAMMING & DATABASES

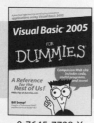

Visual Basic 2005 For Dummies
0-7645-7728-X

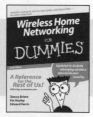

Wireless Home Networking For Dummies
0-471-74940-0

Also available:
- Access 2007 For Dummies 0-470-04612-0
- ASP.NET 2 For Dummies 0-7645-7907-X
- C# 2005 For Dummies 0-7645-9704-3
- Hacking For Dummies 0-470-05235-X
- Hacking Wireless Networks For Dummies 0-7645-9730-2
- Java For Dummies 0-470-08716-1

- Microsoft SQL Server 2005 For Dummies 0-7645-7755-7
- Networking All-in-One Desk Reference For Dummies 0-7645-9939-9
- Preventing Identity Theft For Dummie? 0-7645-7336-5
- Telecom For Dummies 0-471-77085-X
- Visual Studio 2005 All-in-One Desk Reference For Dummies 0-7645-9775-2
- XML For Dummies 0-7645-8845-1